Evolving Concepts in Psychiatry

edited by

PERRY C. TALKINGTON, M.D.
Psychiatrist-in-Chief, Timberlawn Sanitarium

and

CHARLES L. BLOSS, M.D.
Medical Director, Timberlawn Sanitarium

Being Those Papers Presented at a Seminar Commemorating the Fiftieth Anniversary of Timberlawn Psychiatric Center, Dallas, Texas

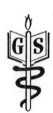

GRUNE & STRATTON / NEW YORK AND LONDON

Contents

Foreword

IN AN ERA when mental disorders became established among those maladies known to have natural causes, and not mystical beginnings, it was fitting that a scientist and teacher such as James J. Terrill develop a penetrating interest in psychiatry. This provided the motivation to disengage himself from the academic world of the University of Texas Medical Branch and establish one of Texas' earliest psychiatric hospitals. In a colonial frame home on the outskirts of Dallas, Dr. Terrill opened a twelve bed hospital incorporated as Timberlawn Sanitarium on June 21, 1917.

Even those who did not know him personally can find the traits of the founder as they are embedded in the current operation and philosophy of Timberlawn and its staff. From the beginning, Dr. Terrill was profoundly convinced of the need to assemble the best possible minds in psychiatry for the benefit of the patient. The first of these was Dr. Guy F. Witt, who became one of the outstanding leaders and clinicians in Texas psychiatry. Dr. Tom H. Cheavens, a later addition, became one of the most energetic and dedicated teachers in Southwestern psychiatry. His untimely death in the Navy during World War II is still felt by those who knew him.

These pioneers of Southwestern psychiatry emphasized the patient as the central figure of the hospital operation and the fact that the patient represented the reason for the existence of the hospital. They felt that all treatment must be based on the fundamental principles and ethics of medical treatment and must embody the most effective known methods. These were not casual men. They exerted a constant effort to improve psychiatric services and facilities for the delivery of psychiatric care. They insisted on the constant recognition of the needs of patients families and the roles of families in the development of the patients disability. They taught forty medical school graduating classes and ever recognized their community responsibility in both civic and civil matters. They insisted on constant improvement of scientific skill by continuous educational exposure not only by the medical staff, but by the members of the treatment team having contact with patients or families. Second only to patient care, Dr. Terrill and his staff insisted on constant research and development of new ideas of diagnosis and treatment. They were always eager to share these experiences with the medical profession.

iv

This program commemorating the Fiftieth Anniversary of Timberlawn Psychiatric Center embodies the best of those principles set forth by these pioneers of psychiatry. It is a fitting memorial to them. We are grateful to those internationally known leaders and educators in psychiatry whose words are recorded in the following pages.

Without the assistance of many people this rewarding meeting could not have been successful. The Chairmen of the Departments of Psychiatry of the Texas Medical Schools have added scientific knowledge and dignity to the program by serving as moderators of sections. Most of all, those in attendance have made the most rewarding contribution by their interest and presence.

Perry C. Talkington, M.D.

Charles L. Bloss, M.D.

Dedication

To the memory of those founders whose principles are reflected in these pages:

James J. Terrill, M.D.
Guy F. Witt, M.D.
Thomas H. Cheavens, M.D.

Contributors

FRANCIS J. BRACELAND, M.D.—Senior Consultant, Institute of Living, Hartford, Connecticut; Editor, American Journal of Psychiatry.

FRANCIS J. GERTY, M.D.—Professor Emeritus of Psychiatry, University of Illinois School of Medicine; Past President of the American Psychiatric Association, Chicago, Illinois.

HENRY W. BROSIN, M.D.—President, American Psychiatric Association; Chairman, Department of Psychiatry, University of Pittsburgh School of Medicine, Pittsburgh, Pennsylvania.

DANA L. FARNSWORTH, M.D.—Henry K. Oliver Professor of Hygiene; Director, University Health Services, Harvard University, Cambridge, Massachusetts.

HERBERT C. MODLIN, M.D.—Director, Division Community Psychiatry, The Menninger Foundation, Topeka, Kansas.

LAWRENCE C. KOLB, M.D.—President-Elect, American Psychiatric Association; Chairman, Department of Psychiatry, College of Physicians and Surgeons, Columbia University, New York, New York.

Psychiatry: Past, Present, Future

FRANCIS J. BRACELAND, M.D.

*"What do you write?" said Gobind. "I write of all matters that
lie within my understanding and of many that do not." "Even
so," said Gobind, "tell them first of those things thou hast seen
and they have seen together. Thus their knowledge will piece
out thy imperfections."*

Life's Handicap . . . Kipling

I, TOO, SPEAK TO YOU of some matters which lie within my understanding
and of some that do not. But we will not worry about imperfections, for this
is a festive occasion, a golden anniversary, a time for celebration, a time for
congratulation to the directors, the staff and all of the personnel of Timberlawn, for they are "the heart of the matter."

Cadmus, a hospital administrator, tells the story of a great university
which once built a fine library. It was a monumental structure of marble
with tall pillars and ornate furnishings. The students and faculty were in-
ordinately proud of it and as they took visitors about they boastfully said,
"This is our new library." Finally, the librarian could stand it no longer and
he put up a big sign which said, "This is not the library—the library is inside."

The same may be said of hospitals. Although modern buildings are
essential and hospitals must have structures that are functional, comfortable and attractive, yet the soul of a hospital—of this hospital—its
essence, is really inside. It is made up of people, skilled, capable,
knowledgeable and dedicated people, and on the happy occasion of
Timberlawn's half century celebration Cadmus' story comes freshly to our
minds.

As a representative of a large number of our colleagues, especially those
from private psychiatric hospitals, I salute you members of the oldest
hospital of your kind in the southwest; in their name and with warmest best
wishes foresee for you an equally productive and rewarding future in your
next half century.

While my subject is *Psychiatry: Past, Present and Future,* I shall not
dwell too long on our past. Although we were nurtured in almshouses, we
really were born in the earliest hospitals ever organized. And in the first two

1

general hospitals organized in our country, provisions were made for psychiatric patients, thus establishing our legitimacy in the new land.

The history of the hospital movement is one of the most absorbing stories in the annals of civilization. Born of elemental needs, the hospital not only has been a tool of society, but also its mirror, faithfully reflecting the religious, philosophic and cultural preoccupations of the time, together with the contemporary level of medical knowledge. The germ of the hospital idea existed even in Babylonian times. The Egyptians, Greeks and Romans had their temples of healing, yet the whole spirit of antiquity toward sickness and misfortune was one of expediency rather than one of compassion. Charity and pity were dispensed by individuals when the spirit moved them.

It was concomitant with the spread of early Christianity that the practice of ministering to human suffering on an extended scale became a guiding principle of society. Believers very early established the rule that each community should assume the responsibility of looking after the sick, the poor, the orphans, the widowed and the infirm, no matter what the state of their reason. Thus, the healing ministry was considered an integral part of community work and an obligation. It is interesting that after all of these centuries, we now are moving back to this same community concept! Truly, "there is nothing new under the sun."

The inception of the modern hospital was under Pope Innocent III and he directed specifically that the mentally ill were to be cared for in each hospital throughout the world that his bishops would establish. Virchow traced the origin of German city hospital back to him and it is a known fact that practically all of the historic British hospitals were related to his era. This heritage was later forgotten as superstition spread and strange concepts of mental disease prevailed. In fact, strange concepts of medical practice arose and the whole field of mental disease became separated from medicine, and hospitals lost sight of their original mission.

I shall not dwell upon our alienation; although there are a few bright spots here and there, in general it is not a pretty story. The heritage of the early voluntary mental hospital in this country, however, is rather a good one and we should keep in mind the fact that it was the private hospitals that kept the treatment of patients on a humane basis in our country when no one seemed to care about them. We can't take time to recount our past glories however, nor can we take time to count our contributions. There are too many contemporary problems pressing upon us which we need to consider and try to forecast our directions.

Even as late as the time Dr. Terrill began his hospital in 1917, psychiatry was quite isolated from its sister disciplines. The myth of incurability of mental disease was abroad in the land; physical medicine was advancing with rapid strides, but our medical brethren seemed to believe only the things they could see, palpate, percuss, auscultate or cut out. There was no time for anything as unscientific as our specialty. That battle is not yet won; twice within the past month I have read in reputable medical journals articles, quite serious, questioning whether psychiatrists really are physicians and whether psychiatry was a medical discipline. Recently, in an opinion before Congress, a member of our own specialty asserted that it would only require a few weeks to teach anyone to use the drugs which are in psychiatry's armamentarium and he thus, by implying that that was all there was to the specialty, called its necessity into question. Thus, the myth of incurability has given rise to the myth of mental disease as a medical problem at all.

But enough of the past. What of the present? Quo Vadis? Where are we and where are we going? We may note at once that our trends, like those of all of medicine, obviously are greatly influenced by the "zeitgeist," or spirit of the times, and influenced not only by rapid scientific advances, but by noteworthy changes in the social and economic scenes of a growing society. Today's goals are tomorrow's outmoded practices. What was envisioned as the millenium by turn-of-the-century leaders in psychiatry, for example, has already been vastly exceeded and in retrospect seems short-sighted, unimaginative and, in some cases, wrong. Once again, we see that change is the present day watchword in psychiatry; the blending of what was worthwhile in the old with the obvious requirement of the new. It vividly recalls to mind Edna St. Vincent Millay's warning that all creatures to survive must adapt to the changing conditions under which they live:

If they can grow new faculties to meet the new necessity, they thrive—otherwise not; the inflexible organism, however much alive today, tomorrow is extinct.[1]

Scientific advances are major forces affecting change in every form of social institution. The extent of this is apparent and understandable when we realize that 5 per cent of all the people and 95 per cent of all the scientists who have ever lived, are alive today. Along with this, and operating in the health field, is the inclusion in our statutes of what has long been a social philosophy, namely, that everyone has the *right* to health care. Financial aid is now available to a large segment of the population without regard to need. This is producing new patterns of distribution and financing of medical care in the United States.

In 1966, the American Hospital Association registered more than 7100 hospitals and these contained 1.7 million beds. Of these, 5700 were non-federal short-term general hospitals accounting for 43 per cent of all beds and 92 per cent of total annual admissions. The other 1400 hospitals, governmental, psychiatric, tuberculosis and others, account for 57 per cent of all beds. Although psychiatric hospitals account for only 7 per cent of the total number of hospitals, they care for 48 per cent of the 1.4 million patients hospitalized on any given day.

Breaking the statistics down a bit further, we note that today the United States has 318 state and local public mental hospitals, 44 government mental hospitals, 165 private psychiatric hospitals and 500 units of ten beds or more in the 5700 community general hospitals. The most surprising thing, however, is that on any one day in the United States more than 250,000 persons visit hospital out-patient departments, for an annual total of more than 90 million. This increase in out-patient visits is one of the startling phenomena of the last few years, and many of these patients have serious emotional problems—just how many, we do not know—and in many localities, the emergency room is now considered an extension of the doctor's office. One other startling figure, and one that should be noted for future reference, is that on any one day there are more than 300,000 persons in educational programs in United States hospitals.

This is the background milieu in which we practice psychiatry today. Little more than a decade ago, there were more than 700,000 patients in state hospitals and nearly an equal number in private, general and other hospitals. Last year, there were only 452,000 patients in state hospitals, a decrease of a quarter of a million, although the population rose nearly 20 per cent in the same period. Iowa furnishes a stellar example of what is happening. Since 1946, the resident state hospital population in Iowa has dropped 75 per cent, from more than 6600 in that year to 1683 in October 1966. Where have these patients gone? They have gone to clinics, halfway houses, mental health centers and institutes. What does all of this mean and why have I presumed to stuff you with statistics? It means that these examples presage our future directions and it behooves us to pay heed to them. Bear with me for a moment while we examine one or two other factors which seem to be pushing us willy-nilly in several directions.

To practice psychiatry, we need, among other things, psychiatrists; and to get psychiatrists we are dependent upon medical manpower. Medical manpower is trained in medical schools and medical schools are, like ourselves, in a vortex at the present time. I think it is safe to say that there is not one medical school in the United States or Canada which is not experimenting with new forms of curricula.

The knowledgeable J. F. McCreary, Dean of the Faculty of Medicine, University of British Columbia, after years of study, recently pointed out to an international assembly the widespread dissatisfaction with the end products of today's medical education and the widespread criticism of medical schools both from within and without the profession. I mention this here for it seems to me that the same factors exerting pressure upon medical educators are also pressing upon practitioners of psychiatry.

In McCreary's opinion, none of the various experimental curricula in medical schools is likely to succeed to any significant degree because the real problem of medical education today is based upon a knowledge explosion and a rapid change in the attitude of people towards medicine and the physician. The physician is trained as though he was to provide his services in the same fashion as he did thirty or forty years ago. Yet the demands made upon him have increased enormously and changed significantly. I can attest to the truth of this. I have been in the practice of medicine for more than one-third of a century and was dean of medicine nearly thirty years ago. The general practitioner oriented system of medicine is not being embraced by medical students, not because of the prospects of hard work or even of finances, but, rather, because of fear of the vast amount of knowledge the man knows he will require if he undertakes to perform this service satisfactorily.

McCreary believes the factors upsetting medical education at present are:

1. The knowledge explosion. The material to be learned is phenomenally great.
2. The changes in the patterns of medical care nationally.
3. The changing economic system and the *right* to receive medical care.
4. The changing attitudes of patients: greater sophistication and, consequently, greater expectations.
5. A change in the popular picture of the physician. Individually, as physicians, we are well thought of; as a group, we have slipped a notch in the affections of the people.

Strangely, however, in all of this psychiatry seems to be faring better than its sister medical disciplines and thus "the stone which the builders rejected" now holds promise of becoming the cornerstone of the new comprehensive medicine which lies before us. Funkenstein, writing in the *American Journal of Psychiatry* one month ago, has this to say:

> An accelerating trend in recent years is that many of the students with the characteristics of clinicians who entered medical school planning to practice by working directly with patients, are now considering psychiatry as a career. They consider medicine in teaching hospitals to be overweighted with science and lacking in the human element. These students see the psychiatrist as the one specialist who still works directly with patients and can afford to be concerned

with the patient as a person. They believe that only in this specialty will they be able to devote themselves to their primary goal of becoming a physician.[2]

This is a turnabout, isn't it? Would it surprise you to know that in a secret straw poll taken in the Junior class of one of the top medical schools in the country two-thirds of the class said they were considering psychiatry. Although this will surely change markedly, it still is noteworthy and psychiatric educators may have their work cut out for them.

How does all of this affect present day psychiatry and what are the trends we are to look for? It is obvious that society is in transition—one might say in a slight convulsion—but as yet there are no definite indications as to what form the new society will assume. Community psychiatry is the present day watchword and, far from being a bandwagon that some have thought it to be, it is a national trend now taken seriously by federal officials, governors and state legislatures. Every state region and town is involved in its own particular fashion. The planning is comprehensive and visualizes cooperation between mental health workers and other members of the caretaking professions and groups. Not all of these agencies are noted for their cooperative spirit nor are they noted for a willingness to give up their often petty jealously guarded prerogatives. If they do cooperate, all will go smoothly; if they do not, the community clinics will deteriorate and just be "other clinics," expensive to run and in competition for scarce manpower. As community clinics grow, attacks will already be mounted upon other pressing problems such as alcoholism, already a scourge. In fact, broad plans are being formulated to attack this problem nationally. Psychiatrists in general practice and those from private as well as state hospitals will have a part to play in these ventures, and intense efforts will be made to prevent state hospitals from becoming repositories or institutions of last resort.

Crisis intervention is the newest psychiatric interest, thus bearing out in practice an old axiom of Erasmus, "It is better to treat at the beginning, etc." Hence, the home and emergency services now in operation. Strangely, general medicine, whose practitioners began in the home and then moved to offices, now is moving into hospitals; while psychiatry, which began in institutions, with its new insights, is moving in a diametrically opposite direction—to offices and into homes.

The Psychiatrist

What is the status of the psychiatrist in today's social and economic upheaval? The citizens are much more sophisticated than ever before and are now interested in the planning of psychiatric services. It is their representatives who appear before legislators in support of mental health budgets, and it is they who make demands upon the psychiatrist for information and help with problems. At present, the psychiatrist is not sure he can meet all of their demands and it is too soon to say whether they represent a real trend or simply a passing interest.

Recently, in addressing a representative group of hospital administrators, Walter Barton recalled that Leo Srole, a medical sociologist, had, several years earlier, characterized psychiatry as "the public's court of last resort" in many psychological dilemmas. He suggested that when ordinary common sense measures failed to solve certain social problems, increasing segments of the population were turning for help to the mental health professions—the experts in "uncommon sense." This is still true and clergymen, judges, educators, industrialists, diplomats, executives, military and laymen now appeal to the psychiatrist for help and advice whenever and wherever they encounter emotional problems or aberrant behavior in the course of their work. Furthermore, some of these groups would like to have a few short courses given so that they may handle similar problems when they arise in the future. This is all a far cry from the situation when Timberlawn began in 1917 and when alienists still were isolated.

Are these directions salutary or not? Are they good or bad? Have we been trained for all of this? Can we advise the present day adolescent about sexual problems? We know the anatomy and physiology and some of the emotional aspects of the situation, but that is only a part of it. What about the pill? To whom will it be given? Unmarried maidens? What about abortion? What knowledge do we have about these problems over and above that of ordinary physicians?

What shall we do as psychiatrists? Shall we stick to our lasts and do the tasks for which we have been trained, or shall we respond to the demands of a society which is pressing for a change, yet does not know what that change will be? In a perceptive article in *Science* in July 1967, Dr. Bryant Wedge examined the question of "Psychiatry in International Affairs." This has been talked of before on a number of occasions. Wedge sees the problems involved and believes that despite them "there is a substantial case for applying psychiatric methods to international affairs." "Clinical psychiatry," Wedge says, "involves the professional application of complex multi-variant analysis and decision making in areas of profound human relationships and in terms of incomplete and inexact information." He feels that psychiatrists have learned to exercise objectivity and compassion with respect to human actions, and that these qualities are desirable in the analysis of international problems, etc., that we may have something of real value to offer in fields of international affairs. "Indeed," he says, "no other profession or discipline is so well prepared by everyday practice."

George Stevenson had put forth comparable opinions in 1941 and suggested, also, that perhaps a way to approach this was conjointly with the behavioral scientists. In answer to these observations, the American Psychiatric Association set up an Ad Hoc Study Group on Dynamic Leadership. Its chairman was the late Dr. Ewen Cameron.

Then where are we going? Does our greatest usefulness and our safety not come from adhering rather strictly to medicine, the discipline which nurtured us? I believe so. We must have a secure base of operations, a harbor we can depend upon when the winds of social change blow this way and that and it does seem that medicine is that harbor, for no matter to what heights man's spirit and intentions may soar, he will still be trammeled with a body.

However, none of this implies that we are to plod on in old-fashioned dogmatic ways, insisting always on fifty minute hours and set rubrics of special methods of treatment laid down decades ago. Two papers at the last annual meeting of the American Psychoanalytic Association exhorted psychoanalysts to take part in community psychiatric efforts. Louis Linn said, "The traditional roles of psychoanalysis in psychotherapy training and research are indispensable in the Era of Community Psychiatry. The psychoanalyst must offer the same skills in relation to the interdisciplinary, consultative process that he has made available over many decades of clinical experience in psychotherapy. Psychoanalysis has not only played a key role in the birth of the Community Psychiatry era, but a continuing major role in bringing this era to its finest fruition."

Bernard Bandler spoke in the same vein when he pointed out that the Psychoanalytic Association grew and prospered when it responded to the challenge of community psychiatry represented by the Second World War. "The psychoanalyst's identity," he said, "was not diluted but enriched. It can again realize its full potential if it responds to the current challenge of community psychiatry." Other writers now deny that "blue collar" workers are impervious to dynamic psychotherapy and thus various groups are enlisting under the contemporary banners.

Walter Barton, in the address previously mentioned, concluded that:

> There is a natural reluctance to sacrifice one of the world's finest medical practice systems to distribute mediocre or second-class medicine to the masses. Some of my colleagues are certain psychiatry must participate in the social evolution and revolution that are today's realities. Not all are agreed. 'What products and services are to be delivered to a vaguely specified consumer?' the others ask. All *are* agreed there must be better distribution of health care to all segments of society.

This puts the problem succinctly. It is my own opinion that medicine and medical education will not work out their problems, nor will psychiatry work out its own until the culture determines the kind of medical care to be furnished and how it is to be furnished. In the meantime, the only things which will advance the cause of all of our disciplines will be a cognizance of change, a malleability rather than case-hardening, and the making of the professions of medicine, and especially psychiatry, life-long educative processes required and supervised by our professional societies.

THE FUTURE

What of the future? When Timberlawn celebrates its 100th anniversary, many of today's psychiatric problems will have been solved, but many others will face you. In our research and advances we seem, as Horace said, to solve one difficulty by raising another (*Litem quod lite resolvit*). We will have traveled far, but man is so complex we will require constant study, patience, good sense and perspective. Oliver Wendell Holmes once observed that "science is a first-rate piece of furniture for man's upper chamber, if he has common sense on the ground floor."

Predictions are hazardous in science for one never knows at what moment something great and new will appear and require a complete revision of our basic concepts and beliefs. Predictions are especially hazardous now for we seem to be on the threshold of a general awakening in all phases of intellectual and scientific life. Some of the portents seem to be visible presently in the new technical advances, so let us take off into fantasy about the future for a few moments.

First, our specialty—long the Cinderella of medicine—will have arrived in state long before Timberlawn's 100th anniversary. The fact that one cannot separate man's psyche from his soma will have percolated through the densest of crania. New fields and specialties will come into being. Nuclear substances will find wider usage. Many present forms of treatment will be superseded.

Illnesses will change their form as mood controlling drugs are perfected. Schizophrenia will be broken down into several congeries of symptoms and no longer will remain a scourge. Genetic control of it is unlikely. Attacks upon metabolic defects may have good results. Drugs may block the abnormal metabolic pathways or unlock the normal ones. Dietary control may even be possible and precipitative situations identified and devoided. Depression will respond quickly to various types of therapy. Behavior disorders will change as the very bright young folks see the uselessness of acting out and the pendulum may even swing to austerity. Addictions may increase for a while as civilization becomes more complicated. Unfortunately, however, man's aggression will not easily be controlled. People who don't agree with us, we still will consider stubborn or wrong just as we do now. Unfortunately—or maybe not so unfortunately—we won't do much toward lengthening man's allotted span of years. His body will continue to get shorter as he ages, but his anecdotes will get longer (as the writer is now demonstrating).

Hospital construction will have changed markedly and, in response to personnel shortages, will be fully automated and numerous labor saving devices used. There will be an increase in circular wards, and television between nursing stations and patients' rooms. This last is not fantasy. It is already in operation. Telemikes now control lights, music, T.V. and calls to nurses' stations. Bathroom facilities will be in every room, close to the beds and blended into the decor of the room. People will help themselves more because of personnel shortages and because psychiatrists have taught them that coddling causes them to regress. Illness thus will lose some, but not all, of its attractiveness for those who would like to be infantalized, but in some instances illness will continue to be a saving grace.

Food will be cooked to the patient's liking, at his own door by mobile food carts; the cooking done by radio waves. The stove will cook steaks in thirty seconds to the patient's order, but, maybe, I had better stop right there. This will be read by so many psychiatrists that this fantasy worries me and someone might report me to my Board of Directors as having excess sludge in my cerebral arteries, or even canaries in my aerial.

Before I close, however, I might add that more and more patients will be admitted to hospitals of some order and the private psychiatric hospitals will have added duties because, of necessity, they will have perfected themselves and additional tasks will be forced upon them. I remind you again that neither private practitioners nor private mental hospitals can ignore the demands for cooperative effort that the community most certainly will urge upon us. To do so might result in our missing a parade that passes only once.

As I leave you, I repeat for you two statements which I believe are apropos. Ours, as you know, is a wonderful discipline and we are fortunate to be part of it. The expertise of the personnel of our hospitals is a precious commodity. Daniel Webster once said:

If we work upon marble, it will perish. If we work upon brass, time will efface it. If we rear temples, they will crumble to dust. But if we work upon man's immortal minds, if we imbue them with high principles, with a just fear of God and love of their fellow men, we engrave upon those tablets something which no time can efface and which will brighten and brighten to all eternity.[3]

This is our mission: to work upon men's immortal minds.

What can we do personally to advance our mission? Sometimes we feel that our efforts are puny and do not count for much, but they really do. Samuel Johnson once commented upon that feeling. He said: "He who wants to do a great deal of good all at once, will never do any."

To his statement I would like to add a codicil. Good is done by degrees. To do the small, the modest thing which lies before us. To realize the spiritual value and irrevocability of our smallest acts. This is to be useful—and the useful and the beautiful are rarely separated.

REFERENCES

1. Millay, E. S. V.: *Conversation at Midnight.*
2. Funkenstein, D. H.: A new breed of psychiatrists. *Amer. J. Psychiat.* 124(2): 226, Aug. 1967.
3. Webster, D.: *Speech* given at Faneuil Hall, Boston, Mass. 1852.

The Private Psychiatric Hospital
I. Phases of Development

FRANCIS J. GERTY, M.D.

DR. TALKINGTON INFORMED ME that the two subjects I am to discuss
are: "The Administration in Psychiatry as Leadership Potential" and "The
Place of the Mental Hospital in Community Health Programs." Dr. Walter
Barton had chosen these titles before he knew that he would have to go to
Russia on a visit to psychiatric facilities there and I have inherited his
assignment. The general outline which the titles suggest will be followed,
noting the principles of administration which apply in making psychiatric
treatment as effective as possible within the confines of the psychiatric
hospital and in the broader field of community mental health service, including the psychiatric unit in the general hospital. The historical perspective and the practical administrative problems will be emphasized with the
private psychiatric hospital as the principal focus of attention. It is fitting to
do this at a period in time when governmental standard setting and financial supports introduce important control effects which tend to obscure
when they do not nullify completely the private and free enterprise role of
standard setting and support in the treatment of human illness. During such
a period of change, leadership becomes a matter of outstanding importance.
Without it, we shall become the victims rather than the beneficiary of an
organizational growth which can ingest us into itself for its own nourish-
ment.

The private psychiatric hospital is now involved in service and administration in a phase of rapidly developing community oriented service.
Its experience has been chiefly with hospital oriented service. No longer is it
enclosed in a nearly impenetrable capsule. There has been an enlargement
of our view about what constitutes hospital service and what is comprised
within the range of psychiatric treatment.

Not only medical, but extremely important socioeconomic and administrative considerations are involved with relation to the developments
that have taken place. The developments themselves are not the result of
theoretical medical design, although they have been shaped by the increase
in knowledge of psychiatric illnesses and the means for treating these illnesses. They are a result of the pressure to satisfy needs now envisioned on

12

a larger scale than ever before and of a more pressing immediacy. A hospital-like institution is an old agency for treatment of patients with psychiatric disorders, but private psychiatric service to patients in hospitals, especially in urban areas, is quite different from what it used to be. The phasing of the development through which change has been effected is worthy of review.

PHASE I—THE ASYLUM AND LUNACY (*frankly termed "asylum" and frankly termed "lunacy"*)

In this stage of development, there was strong tendency, which still exists, to distinguish between "insanity" and "nervousness," but insanity received the greater share of public and medical attention. If there was not a tacit denial of the existence of nonpsychotic mental illness, there was scanty recognition of its importance. The asylums were built for the care of lunatic patients. They were regarded as retreats, kinds of mental penitentiaries furnishing refuges from an unaccepting society, and in the beginning were not primarily medically oriented. Those medical practitioners who became interested in the asylums and retreats favored the idea of isolation of the patient from the community in order to benefit the patient, a view justified at the time because of the nature of the cases received and the condition and resources of society for dealing with them. The general hospital then had not developed as the community treatment resource we now know. Most medical treatment was practiced in the home. Organized nurse training had not yet appeared. There was little understanding of the nature of infection or of antisepsis and asepsis. Anesthesia was still in its infancy in 1850. The tremendous advances in knowledge concerning these things chiefly affected physical treatment in the general hospital. The impact of advance in the knowledge of psychiatry was to come later, but the psychotic mental patient had to be cared for by the best means known—the asylum. The more extreme manifestations o f what we now classify as psychoneurosis were medical curiosities such as could be seen in the hysterical cases of Charcot's Clinic. For the most part nervousness, the "vapors," hypochondria and "declines" that were not definitely determined to be physical covered this range of cases. The writings of Bright, Cheyne and Burton referred particularly to the borderline group of illnesses lying between melancholy states and hypochondriasis. Theoretical and practical knowledge about this realm of medicine was rudimentary. For reasons already mentioned, the aid of modern-type hospital facilities for exploration of means of treatment were not available. The problem of psychoneurotic illness was there. It was not perceived as we now perceive

it, largely because attention was focused upon developing facilities to take
care of the seemingly more pressing problems of insanity. The development
of public and private asylums became the vogue. The idea of isolation
prevailed in the asylums and together with unwieldy expansion compounded the difficulties that come from eliminating the community as an
alert monitor of the treatment institutions which serve it.

PHASE II—THE SANITARIUMS AND "NERVOUS EXHAUSTION"

The leading American neuropsychiatrist from 1870 to 1914 was S. Weir
Mitchell, a critic of isolationism and an advocate of rest cure institutions
for patients with nervous exhaustion. The sanitarium rather than an asylum
or a retreat became the in-patient service for neurotic patients who were
now viewed as suffering from nervous exhaustion. New terms were added
to hysteria and hypochondriasis—neurasthenia, psychasthenia and others.
Tuke's historically important dictionary of psychological medicine published
in 1892 gives an account of views then held. "The systematic treatment of
functional neuroses until late years has been the despair of physicians. No
one will contest this statement who will reflect on his experience of such
cases. To have a systematized, a scientific and rational means of dealing
with such illness is no slight achievement and constitutes one of the greatest
gains to practical medicine of which the present generation can boast. This
we owe to the sagacity and intimate knowledge of this form of disease
possessed by S. Weir Mitchell of Philadelphia, by whose name the method
of the systematic treatment is very generally known." The guide for case
selection for treatment in rest cure institutions was given as follows:
"nervous exhaustion," neurasthenia as described by Beard in 1868, hysteria
and narcosis (meaning drug addictions). Specifically excluded were two
types of mental illness: what was called "real mental illness"—i.e.,
psychotic—and one other type, the overfed and selfish neurotic. The chief
elements of the treatment were these: (1) removal from home and community influences (again isolation); (2) massage and electricity to encourage catabolic metabolism as a stimulus to active anabolic metabolism;
(3) overfeeding on a systematic plan under medical supervision. As the
system developed, hydrotherapy was used, and the usual medicinal methods
then in use for purposes of sedation and stimulation were also employed.

It is stated that Freud in his earlier work in Vienna used a modified form
of rest cure management for some of his patients. The institutions using
Mitchell's method with several modifications that were related to it were
usually called sanitariums. Specialized forms of sanataria such as liquor
and narcotic cures appeared. There were a great many of these sanitaria in

the last half of the 19th century and the early decades of the 20th century. Sometimes their administration was related to that of an adjoining service for psychotic patients, commonly in a separate division of service. Sacred Heart Sanitarium and St. Mary's Hill, Milwaukee, represent this type of coverage of the range of mental illness. It is to be noted that in both the asylums and the sanitariums, isolation was a requisite and the return to the community was determined by the patient's restoration to a state of health, particularly "energy storage," which would enable him to cope with his environment more satisfactorily. In the isolation, there was implicit acknowledgement of the fact that interpersonal relationships of the patient played a part in causation and presumably in remedy. However, systematic exploration of the psychodynamics of origin and of remedy through a psychotherapy based on this exploration was not part of the system, at least in the beginning. The principle followed was much more that of recharging a run down battery.

While Mitchell was aware of the importance of interpersonal relationships and some of their sexual aspects, he gave his attention chiefly to the restoration of the physical vitality and energy of the patient. Thorough exploration for any trace of causation in the area of sex was rejected by him or at least not approached with an open mind. His son-in-law, Dr. Cadwalader, relates that Mitchell threw one of Freud's books into the fireplace remarking, "Where did this filthy thing come from?" From the present day psychiatrist's viewpoint, Mitchell's greatest contribution to modern psychiatry was what Dr. John Whitehorn terms his historic scolding of psychiatrists and psychiatric practices given in the address he delivered before the American Psychiatric Association in 1894. He was at that time America's foremost neuropsychiatrist and had warned when invited to speak that he would do so in criticism rather than in compliment. In preparation, he gathered information by the familiar questionnaire method from a number of eminent physicians, William Osler and John Billings among them. He criticized the isolationism of the alienists, their smugness, lack of progress in their scientific approach, and, in general, their isolation from the rest of medicine in their preoccupation with internal details of administration instead. He recommended less of isolation from the medical profession and the community, better training of permanent assistants with attention given to acquiring knowledge of psychology and neuropathology. Especially, he asked for a higher quality of nursing, and then emphasized *"demand of your people original report or product of some kind."*

There was much that was good in Mitchell's criticism, but it had its weaknesses. It did not set the pattern which psychiatric research was to follow. While he suggested neurological and environmental studies, he did not foresee that the productive investigation would concern interpersonal relationships through the psychological and psychoanalytical approach stimulated by Freud and his followers and now by much more refined neurological and recording methods. Even though the operations of both the asylums and the sanitaria were predicated on the principle of temporary isolation of the patient, Mitchell did not favor isolation of the physician and other professionals working in those institutions from the realities which are encountered in the stream of life. He saw the physician as a special servant of mankind who somehow lost caste and deteriorated in knowledge when isolated in an asylum with his patients. In this he was right. He did not as fully and clearly discern the effect of indefinite isolation on the patient, nor did he perceive the nature and potency of the energies which flow over the pathways of association between individuals with their resultant effects in the production of illness and the possibility of using them for the relief of illness.

PHASE III—PRIVATE PRACTICE AND CLINIC SERVICE FOR AMBULATORY PSYCHIATRIC PATIENTS.

Private practice of neurology in the last half of the 19th century included psychiatry in a minor subspecialty position. The remedies used were medicines and electric stimulation, and, for psychological approach, chiefly persuasion and suggestion. Sometimes hypnotism was employed and sometimes authoritative direction. Gradually a change came about during the 20th century. The influence of the work of Freud and his followers increased greatly from the turn of the century through World War II. A new kind of private practice appeared with psychiatry in the position of an independent specialty. A medical directory for Chicago for 1923 lists remarkably few physicians as specializing exclusively in psychiatry. Today there are some 15,000 psychiatrists who are members of the American Psychiatric Association compared to less than a thousand in that year.

The influence of Freud's psychoanalysis was not alone responsible for the change. The psychobiological school of Adolf Meyer insisted upon a comprehensive view of all factors entering into disturbed behavior. Meyer proposed methods of investigating life histories of patients in a much more searching way than had hitherto been the practice. Meyer's concept of the ergasias is a sound one which is generally accepted in principle, although his terminology has fallen into disuse. His views of a need for community centering of the practice of psychiatry were given many years before such ideas gained general acceptance. It was largely due to his insistence that inclusion of psychiatry in the curriculum of the medical school finally became obligatory. Training and research institutes attached to the medical college hospitals and the state hospital systems led to the development of the pattern of out-patient clinics. Also, the importance of child psychiatry was emphasized by William Healey, under whose influence the first child psychiatry clinic was established as the Institute for Juvenile Research in Chicago.

All these undertakings had their effect in putting the private practice of psychiatry on a firm foundation and in an independent position. There was now a very different approach to the treatment of the kinds of disorders that are spoken of as psychoneuroses, neurotic character disorders and psychosomatic disorders. The ground was prepared for the newly gained knowledge of psychiatry to move towards the hospitals, both the general hospitals and the public and private institutions which had been known as asylums and sanitariums. Mental illness was no longer synonomous with insanity.

PHASE IV—MODERN PSYCHIATRY (A NEW ORIENTATION, PSYCHIATRICALLY AND ADMINISTRATIVELY).

From the vantage point of private practice, a community-centered practice we must remember, the psychiatrist, having escaped from institutional isolation has begun to take an active part in community hospital service as well as office practice. There has also been an effect from this on public hospital systems. In Illinois and elsewhere, zone-centered hospitals and clinics are struggling through their initial difficult stages of development. The larger and better known private general hospitals now almost invariably have departments of psychiatry with in-patient units. The private sanitariums of thirty years ago now usually employ means and methods of operation that enable them to be classified as hospitals. Inspecting agencies and insurance against cost of illness have contributed to making this change. Community needs have resulted in establishment of many new private psychiatric hospitals. Meeting these needs will require that psychiatrists, administrative personnel of hospitals, boards of directors and, in the case of proprietary hospitals, owners must find means for providing hospital care for patients that is psychiatrically oriented and, in hospital programming of treatment, will truly back up and strengthen the individual therapy contribution of the psychiatrist. Oversimplified separation of insanity from functional nervous disorder represents a dichotomy of ideas which can only exist by ignoring the fact that body and mind have a continuity of relationships and that this functional continuity also involves many environmental factors which are important in preserving health or producing illness in the total personality. This does not mean that separate organs of the body, separate aspects of psychological functions, or separate diseases or disorders are not entitled to separate consideration. It does mean that this separate consideration must always be given with an over-all view that perceives the unifying purposes which make the whole individual more than the sum of its parts and sees that individual as living in his environmental setting.

It is not a rhetorical question when we ask, "What does this have to do with hospital treatment of mentally ill patients, or, for that matter, of all patients who may happen to be in hospitals?" The practical side of hospital management is involved in a very real way when we use the psychiatrically oriented approach. The pressures of social discomfort connected with the illness of the patient play their part in bringing the patient to our attention. A real and adequate understanding of the implications of the several interrelationships involved must come to influence the mechanized structure of hospital facilities and their administration if the treatment of the patient is to accomplish the most that can be expected of it.

At this time, it may be well to note that the relationship of administration to rendering psychiatric service has been subject to reinspection and action by the Executive Committee of the American Psychiatric Association. The committee approved a change of name for the APA Committee on Certification of Mental Health Administrators to Committee on Certification in Administrative Psychiatry. The Executive Committee which approved this change in title referred back to the Committee on Certification for further recommendation the proposal for the establishment of two groups of applicants for certification, hospital based administrators and community health administrators, with recommendation that some attempt be made which might effect a unified psychiatric examination test for the applicants. Undoubtedly this is the result of the tendency which developed to set up different types of administration from those which have been more or less standard and traditional in psychiatric circles and which originated when the psychiatric hospital was an institution considerably isolated from the communities from which its patients had come.

In the supplementary mailing of the APA Hospital and Community Psychiatry Service recently, there was distributed a paper on the Professional in Mental Hospital Administration. The introduction specifies that what is being discussed is a professional role of a hospital business administrator, and three models of organization are presented. No pointed conclusions are reached. These points do appear: The field of psychiatric service is changing. There is a manpower shortage, especially among professional psychiatrists for hospital work. The indications are that many nonpsychiatric administrators could be found to enter the field. Finally, there is a paucity of research in the whole subject of mental health administration.

I might discuss administration of psychiatric service in several different settings—in the public psychiatric hospital and the system of which it is a part; in the psychiatric unit of the general hospital and the somewhat related medical or university hospital; in the private psychiatric hospital, proprietary and nonprofit; in the community mental health services, chiefly out-patient at present; and in their relation to health services generally. But this would introduce so many aspects of the subject of administration that there would be pointless scattering of emphasis. Therefore, only one subject will receive principal attention: the private psychiatric hospital, proprietary and nonproprietary, considered as a part of community mental health services.

The Mental Status Examination Aided by Microanalysis of Sound Film

HENRY W. BROSIN, M.D.

INTRODUCTION

I WANT TO EXPRESS my appreciation for the privilege of participating in the Fiftieth Anniversary Seminar of Timberlawn Psychiatric Center; the Board of Directors, officers and staff of Timberlawn are to be congratulated for their successful creation of a health unit devoted to the care of distressed people, particularly because it operates within the framework of the free enterprise system and thus preserves many of the best elements of that system. In our current national efforts to extend better health care to all people, we can look to Timberlawn and other similar institutions for guidance and comparative practices, insofar as they are applicable, to help us design better patterns of medical care in the large public networks. The vigorous efforts to furnish ever large quantities of service are justified because the need is very great, but we must *not* lose sight of the equally urgent needs of improved quality, and of teaching and research. The latter are essential for the preservation and enhancement of those human values which we cherish most: individuality, freedom of choice, opportunity for growth, and the dignity of the individual. It is unfortunate that in discussions of patterns of medical practice in recent years we seldom hear of these issues apart from political and economic issues, and yet we must not neglect the dominance of human values in the long run just because medical economics and vital political necessities are in the forefront at this time. It is our good fortune that Timberlawn and similar psychiatric centers have the potentiality for furnishing leadership in the improved practice of medicine, and in originating and developing new methods of care because they have greater freedom for experimentation. It is with this hope that we look forward toward their next half-century of achievement.

THE BASIC IMPORTANCE OF DESCRIPTION: THE PSYCHIATRIC HISTORY, PSYCHIATRIC INTERVIEW AND SPECIAL EXAMINATIONS.

There is no need for me to justify to this audience of psychiatrists the reasons for training ourselves to become better observers and recorders of the interaction between psychiatrists and their patients. All of our teachers in the early part of the century, including Kraepelin, Bleuler, Freud and Adolf Meyer, by eloquent precept and concrete example taught their students that these were the fundamental tools of the psychiatrist in order to understand the phenomena under consideration. We moved over the years from the more static question-and-answer type of history taking to the more dynamic open-ended inquiries in which the patient was given encouragement, under guidance by skilled questioners, to speak much more freely about his feelings and about his own view of his internal and external problems, and thus provide the physician with a rich narrative which gave clues to the disordered relations troubling the patient. Unfortunately, many psychiatrists, for various reasons, after 1945 only paid lip service to sound description in the belief they were learning all they needed to know by studying motivational themes as they appeared in the lexical (verbal) productions of the patient. It is curious that one justification for this was the psychoanalytic model, yet Freud, Ferenczi, Wilhelm Reich, together with leaders such as Ives Hendrick, L. S. Kubie and many others, strongly supported the need for better description as the road to better understanding, and also to scientific verification. Without good records, particularly those which can be reviewed by multiple observers so comparisons can be made, there is no good way to gain consensus on many important issues. Clinicians, like many social scientists, cannot easily replicate the complex systems with which they work. Control series are similarly not easily available if one works in depth, although we might do better if we tried harder and had better resources.

There are many reasons why sound-film recording of interviewing could be of advantage to psychiatrists as clinicians, investigators and educators at many levels. I cannot survey these areas now, even though this is an attractive prospect, and will limit myself to only one special field of investigation, namely the microanalysis of a very few samples of linguistic and kinesic (body-motion) studies which illustrate the potentialities available to the investigator. I want to stress the fact that the amount of time necessary for viewing sound film at the microlevel, not to mention special training, skills and motivation, do not make these methods attractive or easily available to a hard working clinician at this stage of development. It is hoped that, if these methods become sufficiently useful for differential diagnosis and for other comparative studies, specialists will appear who can be of genuine aid to other clinical investigators and even to therapists wanting an opinion about obscure problems.

THE BACKGROUND HISTORY OF THIS PROJECT: THE NATURAL HISTORY OF AN INTERVIEW AND OTHERS.

Nineteenth century psychiatrists defined psychiatry as dealing with disorders of thinking, feeling and acting, and there are ample references to the manner in which a patient spoke or moved which was significant in the diagnosis. This is particularly true of the disorders, incongruities and dyssynchronies of pieces of behavior, especially in speech sequences or in body motions, and it is here that we can give examples that are not usually recorded, but that undoubtedly are perceived subliminally and form a part of the data utilized by the clinician in his evaluations. I have defined "intuition," as it is customarily applied to a knowledgeable clinician, as unverbalized information which has been perceived subliminally. The dictionary definition of intuition is "The power of knowing, or the knowledge obtained, without recourse to inference or reasoning; innate or instinctive knowledge."[31] I believe that what we call intuitive people are those whose subliminal perceptions are available for inferences, and will try to show how these perceptions can be made more available by observing sound-film more minutely.

Philosophers and poets have for generations made reference to the fact that written words are inadequate vehicles for expressing emotions. Spinoza probably deserves credit for being among the first to be explicit about human behavior as a part of all natural law, and showing keen insight in emotional processes and what we call psychodynamics.[30] Our story may well begin with Darwin and Freud and their pupils. Many psychoanalysts since Freud have been interested in the related topics of the evolution of behavior including emotions and language, and the properties of language and body motion in communication systems. Knapp points out that Darwin was an intellectual ancestor to Freud in "the psychologic sphere of the unitary view" of man, and it is likely that many other similarities can be found, as pointed out by numerous authors including S. Bernfeld, E. Erikson, Lucille B. Ritvo and Lili Peller.[1,2,10,24,30]

Coming from the humanities, including psychology and anthropology, and reinforced by Adolf Meyer's belief in the behavioral sciences, including linguistics and anthropology, I was most receptive to Freud's view of training for psychoanalysis: "It must include elements from the mental sciences, from psychology, the history of civilization and sociology, as well as from anatomy, biology and the study of evolution."[13,19]

Freud's "Psychopathology of Everyday Life" (1901, Standard Edition Vol. 6, 1960) and "Jokes and their Relation to the Unconscious" (1905, Standard Edition Vol. 8, 1960) have provided ample material in addition to dream analysis that unconscious processes are present in daily transactions, and the earlier work has always seemed to me to be a good textbook for clinicians and students of human interaction. Among many other excellent examples, I will mention one which Freud used in "Dora" in order to explain the true nature of "symptomatic acts."[12]

> I give the name of symptomatic acts to those acts which people perform, as we say, automatically, unconsciously, without attending to them, or as if in a moment of distraction. They are actions to which people would like to deny any significance, and which, if questioned about them, they would explain as being indifferent and accidental. Closer observation, however, will show that these actions, about which consciousness knows nothing or wishes to know nothing, in fact gives expression to unconscious thoughts and impulses, and are therefore most valuable and instructive as being manifestations of the unconscious which have been able to come to the surface. There are two sorts of conscious attitudes possible towards these symptomatic acts. If we can ascribe inconspicuous motives to them we recognize their existence; but if no such pretext can be found for conscious use we usually fail altogether to notice that we have performed them.
>
> But a justification of this kind [conscious rationalization] does not dismiss the possibility of the action in question having an unconscious origin. Though on the other hand the existence of such an origin and the meaning attributed to the act cannot be conclusively established. We must content ourselves with recording the fact that such a meaning fits in quite extraordinarily well with the situation as a whole and with the programme laid down by the unconscious. (Man muss sich begnügen zu konstatieren, dass ein solcher Sinn in der Tagesordnung des Unbewussten ganz ausgezeichnet hineinpasst.)
>
> There is a great deal of symbolism of this kind in life, but as a rule we pass it by without heeding it. When I set myself the task of bringing to light what human beings keep hidden within them, not by the compelling power of hypnosis, but by observing what they say and what they show, I thought the task was a harder one than it really is. He that has eyes to see and ears to hear may convince himself that no mortal can keep a secret. If his lips are silent, he chatters with his fingertips; betrayal oozes out of him at every pore. And thus the task of making conscious the most hidden recesses of the mind is one which it is quite possible to accomplish.

Knapp has written a survey of the growing interest in communication (1963) and I need not attempt to repeat here the names of many workers on the long road of an interest in the study of the development of language as a social system from Plato, Spinoza, Sir William Jones (1746-94), Darwin and Nietzsche, to mention only a very few of the more well-known names who preceded the more recent families of students of interest to us, particularly the linguist-anthropologists Edward Sapir (1884-1939), who saw clearly during the 1920's the relations between language as a social system and psychiatry, including unconscious factors, and Kenneth L. Pike, who developed a usable method for recording variations in spoken language in 1942 and has since elaborated upon language as an organized hierarchal, highly structured, ongoing, continuous system as a component of other social system.[22,23,25]

The works of Ferenczi and Wilhelm Reich (1933) are well known; other psychoanalysts, such as M. Nina Searl (1933), E. Kris (1939), L. Rangell (1954), R. Spitz (1957), S. S. Feldman (1959) and Anna Freud also discussed expressive behavior as contrasted with verbal behavior. While dozens of other psychoanalysts could be added to the list, I agree with Knapp that T. Braatøy (1954) and Felix Deutsch (1952, 1959) were the only ones who saw the potentials of dealing systematically with expressive behavior or body motions, posture and gestures in the clinical situation.[4,8,9]

At this level of concepts and methods, I do not have anything new to offer. My major goal is to present a few pieces of data which illustrate the possibilities of recording a few dimensions of human behavior not energetically pursued by clinicians by the use of sound film. The emphasis is totally upon the method, and not upon interpretations which will appear as secondary products—these may become more interesting and valuable if we learn to handle the basic recording with greater speed and efficiency.

I would like to insert a footnote inquiry of historical interest. What would be the present status of film recording if Freud had approved of Karl Abraham's proposal (with Hanns Sachs) in 1925? Did Dr. Felix Deutsch, who was a personal physician to Freud for some time (circa 1923), have any writings on the subject? Of course, his film was to be an expository commercial enterprise, and not a scientific project.[11]

I want to give credit to my colleagues, the late Dr. Frieda Fromm-Reichmann, the linguists Professor Norman A. McQuown (University of Chicago), Professor Charles Hockett (Cornell University) and Professor R. L. Birdwhistell (Temple University), and Mr. Gregory Bateson (now in Hawaii), who helped my understanding of many aspects of linguistics, particularly from the viewpoint of cultural anthropology. The first three named and myself agreed in December, 1955, to study the formal properties of language and body motion at the level of microanalysis in order to better understand the myriad rapid signals and messages which occur when two people speak to one another. Bateson provided films and much information, as did Birdwhistell during the summer of 1956 and since. We were also helped in linguistic analyses by two well-known authorities, Professors George L. Trager and Henry L. Smith, Jr., who were then in Buffalo during 1957-1959. The results of this long collaboration will be published in book form, probably in 1969, in a monograph entitled *The Natural History of an Interview*, edited by Norman A. McQuown. It will have extensive examples of linguistic and kinesic analysis of small segments of human interaction.

Most psychoanalysts, whatever their degree of interest, are apt to view the task of microanalysis of film as not *adding* much new information because clinical treatment interviews are so prolonged and human communication so abundantly redundant that they have no need for it. I thoroughly agree with the redundancy position. I also agree that microanalysis is not suited for clinical use at the present stage of technical development because of the enormous amount of time, energy and special skills required. There are also many technical difficulties regarding the introduction of a third element, the camera, into the privacy of the psychoanalytic transference; the distortions introduced by a black and white two-dimensional picture; and many others. However, I think it might be worthwhile to pursue this method to see if there are any potentials for use at the research level. At the very least, films, no matter how crude, are permanent records which could be examined by multiple observers over time, and thus give us a beginning for comparative and longitudinal studies. It is a pleasure to report that there are now many psychoanalysts more tolerant of this prospect than in former years in spite of the many technical barriers to progress. If one recalls the early history of the numerous difficulties surrounding the introduction of instrumentation such as thermometry and the use of the microscope, we might be more tolerant of sound films as a relatively new tool for clinical investigation. Many of these problems are discussed by several authors in *Methods of Research in Psychotherapy*, edited by L. A. Gottschalk and A. H. Auerbach.[16] The essay, "An Experiment in Filmed Psychotherapy," by Paul Bergman is notable for its skillful management of many of the objections cited.[16, pp. 35-49]

I am also sure that use could be made of sound films in the teaching of general psychiatry and family dynamics at the level of gross interaction, but that is beyond the scope of this article.

EXPERIENCE OF H. SARLES, E. J. CHARNY, F. F. LOEB AND W. S. CONDON

Keeping in mind the thesis that the history of a science is the history of its technology, and hoping to find ways in which better recording by means of sound film might improve our data and insights, workers at Pittsburgh attempted several methods of observing and correlating data. We knew that there were many technical barriers, that truly new information might be rare, and that the results might eventually be rewarding only to an

DISTANCE OF PITCH RISE (R) DECREASES OVER THE SENTENCE (ɑ ɑ ɑ ɑ ɑ)

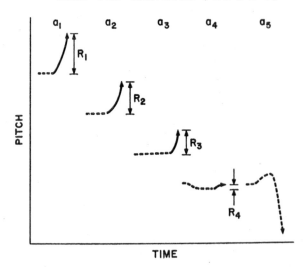

FIG. 1 (*Sarles*).

obsessional collector with an excessive preoccupation with small details. On the other hand was the pleasure derived from being able to document even relatively simple relations with greater precision and clarity than ever before. Even though current methods and results are crude, we were encouraged by the belief that refinements are inevitable and that unexpected applications would probably appear which would justify the expenditure of large amounts of energy.

For example, Sarles, a linguist-anthropologist, using a film at "double-slow motion" (48 frames per second), found a way to illustrate simply with many different subjects that our total sentences to come are characteristically programmed in advance in straightforward short unambiguous statements. Figures 1, 2, 3 and 4 illustrate his finding that pitch and stress are predetermined in successive elements, particularly after the first element or two.[26] Figure 4 shows three lexical items which are differentiated by the use of pitch and stress, e.g., to differentiate a man who keeps a lighthouse from a woman who is an underweight housekeeper.

Charny, a psychoanalytically trained psychiatrist, utilizing films made in 1956 by Bateson of a therapeutic interview of 33 minutes duration found consistent consonant postural behavior or postural harmony, in keeping with the changes in the lexical productions of both. Analyzing the postural configurations of the patient and the therapist into categories named con-

DISTANCE (D) FROM INITIAL PITCH TO ONSET OF PITCH RISE INCREASES FROM WORD TO WORD

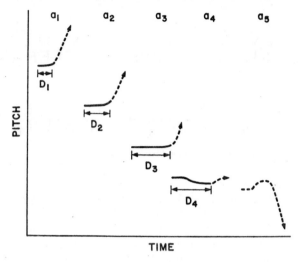

FIG. 2 (*Sarles*).

INITIAL PITCH OF WORDS IS LOWER (P) THAN INITIAL PITCH OF PRECEDING WORD

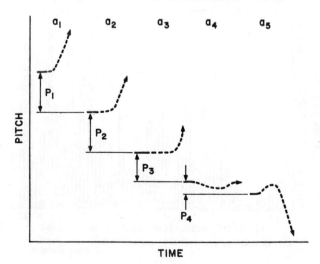

FIG. 3 (*Sarles*).

2 /   1 \   ∧   ∪ 1
I.   LIGHT   HOUSE   KEEPER #

2 \   3 /   \   ∪ 1
2.   LIGHT   HOUSE   KEEPER #

2 ∧   3 /   1 \   ∪ 1
3.   LIGHT | HOUSE   KEEPER #

FIG. 4 (*Sarles*).

gruent and noncongruent, Charny also examined the vocal behavior with each of the postural types both structurally and thematically. He found that the vocal correlates of congruent posture "were consistently positive, interpersonal, specific, and bound to the therapeutic situation, whereas those occurring with noncongruent configurations were more self-oriented, negational, and nonspecific, and tended to be self-contradictory and nonreferenced."[6]

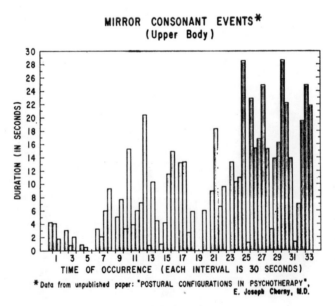

MIRROR CONSONANT EVENTS*
(Upper Body)

* Data from unpublished paper: "POSTURAL CONFIGURATIONS IN PSYCHOTHERAPY",
E. Joseph Charny, M.D.

FIG. 5 (*Charny*).

SUMMARY OF DATA - UPPER BODY CONSONANCE*
DISTRIBUTIONAL DATA

	MIRROR CONSONANT PERIODS	IDENTICAL CONSONANT PERIODS	NON−CONSONANT PERIODS
DURATION	0.4 TO .44.5 SECS. INCREASES AS INTERVIEW PROGRESSES	0.4 TO 3.7 SECS. VARIABLE	0.4 TO 92.2 SECS. DECREASES AS INTERVIEW PROGRESSES
FREQUENCY	INCREASES AS INTERVIEW PROGRESSES	DECREASES AS INTERVIEW PROGRESSES	DECREASES AS INTERVIEW PROGRESSES
PERCENTAGE OF TOTAL TIME	29 % (9 MINS. 24 SECS.)	2 % (30 SECS.)	69 % (23 MINS. 23 SECS.)

* DATA FROM UNPUBLISHED PAPER: "POSTURAL CONFIGURATIONS IN PSYCHOTHERAPY", E. JOSEPH CHARNY, M.D.

FIG. 6 (Charny).

Charny concludes that congruent postural configurations in these situations are behavioral indicators of rapport, and therefore may be of value in
analysis of behavior. Similar findings cited by Charny have been published
by A. E. Scheflen, formerly of the Temple University Department of
Psychiatry and the Eastern Pennsylvania Psychiatric Institute and now at
Downstate University, New York.[28]

Loeb and Condon, using the same film described above, studied the interactions of the patient and therapist at the levels of lexical, linguistic and
kinesic (body motion) activity. In this and numerous other films they found
that identifiable linguistic and kinesic units tended to occur in specific lexical and/or "meaning class" contexts. Parenthetically, I should mention

SUMMARY OF DATA - UPPER BODY CONSONANCE*
CONTENT CORRELATES

MIRROR CONSONANT PERIODS	INTERVIEW STARTS AND ENDS IN MIRROR CONSONANT POSTURE FOUR OF FIVE UTTERANCES BY THERAPIST OCCUR DURING MIRROR CONSONANT PERIODS
IDENTICAL CONSONANT PERIODS	PATIENT'S NARRATIVE REFLECTS CONTENT PATTERN OF INTERVIEW AS A WHOLE
NON - CONSONANT PERIODS	PATIENT'S NARRATIVE SUMMARIZES EVENTS OF PREVIOUS DAY

*DATA FROM UNPUBLISHED PAPER: "POSTURAL CONFIGURATIONS IN PSYCHOTHERAPY", E. JOSEPH CHARNY, M.D.

FIG. 7 (Charny).

SUMMARY OF DATA - UPPER BODY CONSONANCE *
LEXICAL CORRELATES

MEANING- WORD CLASSES	MIRROR CONSONANT PERIODS	IDENTICAL CONSONANT PERIODS	NON-CONSONANT PERIODS
LOCATIVE	INFREQUENT NON-SPECIFIC	NONE	FREQUENT SPECIFIC
TEMPORAL	FREQUENT SPECIFIC	INFREQUENT NON-SPECIFIC	INFREQUENT
SUBJECTIVE	PRONOUN "I" NON-SPECIFIC PRONOUNS	SPECIFIC	VARIABLE
VERBAL	NEGATIVE OR NON-ACTION REFLEXIVE	ACTION AND NON-ACTION	VARIABLE

*DATA FROM UNPUBLISHED PAPER: "POSTURAL CONFIGURATIONS IN PSYCHOTHERAPY", E. JOSEPH CHARNY, M.D.

FIG. 8 (*Charny*).

that Condon has considerable evidence for which he is seeking publication that basically the lexical-linguistic-kinesic components are not three separate systems in a well integrated larger system, but rather are a unitary whole or gestalt. Breakdowns in the larger and smaller systems will be seen in examples from patients suffering from aphasia, stuttering and schizophrenia.

Loeb isolated one gesture, called "S_2," which consists of a specific pattern of movements which resembles a grasping movement. This gesture occurs with the words "in," "out" or "off" and in every case with the meaning class "something or someone getting 'off' ('out') or away from the patient or her mind," or with the meaning class "someone or something getting 'in' close to her or her mind."

The identical pattern was identified in another film of the same patient in a very different context, and also in another film where a psychiatrist from a different subculture uses the same gesture in the same meaning class. Because such differences in the lexical context may be either regional or characterologic, more comparisons, particularly crosscultural ones, must be done before generalizations are in order. Loeb offers the hypothesis that this gesture and others similar to it may be related to various manifestations of the grasp reflex seen in human infants, and in other mammals, such as cats and dogs, and may be a signal revealing unconscious activity which has remained remarkably free from modification by experience or ego control.

Loeb describes an "expression system" as an abstract category which stands for a certain class of behaviors such as speech, sounds, movements, visceral activity.[18] (This is an expansion of Gleason's linguistic terminology.) The "content system" refers to ". . . the subject of the discourse," "ideas, . . . the things man reacts to and tries to convey to his fellows."[15] Using the psychoanalytic model which has proved so useful in understanding dreams, hypnosis, neurosis, psychosis, slips, parapraxis, wit, Loeb has further divided the structural linguistic content system of Gleason into two major subsystems. The first is the preconscious content system which includes the conventional conscious content system, and an unconscious content system. These distinctions follow Freud's suggestions in *The Ego and the Id* (1923) without any topographical implications, but are strictly descriptive; nor do they correspond to the psychic agencies which oppose each other in mental conflicts.[18] Loeb stresses Freud's insight that ". . . the unconscious of one human being can react upon that of another, without passing through the conscious.[14, p. 194]

In the same 33 minute film mentioned earlier, Loeb identifies eighteen fist-like movements (expressive system) within ten separate contexts (preconscious content system). The basic concept "anger" occurred overtly only in seven of the eighteen fist-like movements: There were two lexical expressions denoting anger without the fist, but since the left hand was not visible in these two scenes, it could not be determined whether a fist-like movement was present or not. The remaining eleven fist-like movements occurred in seven lexical categories which refer to "frustration" or "being frustrated in her work to contact her therapist during the few days prior to

OCCURRENCES OF "OFF" OR "OUT" WITH S2

1. (974)₁ THINKING THAT THIS (PHENOBARBITAL) WOULD GET 'EM (BILLY) OFF TO SLEEP RIGHT AWAY

2. (1063)₁ HE (BILLY) WAS BEING WAS JUS' COMPLETELY OUT

3. (1306)₁ YOU CAN'T TELL HER (FRIEND II) THAT BECAUSE SHE WOULDN'T HAVE SENSE ENOUGH TO SEE IT AN' TO GET HER OFF ON ANOTHER GREAT LONG DISSERTATION

4. (1331)₁ SHE (FRIEND II) WOULDN'T DO ANYTHING AN' JUST LYING RIGHT OUT IN THE SUN

5. (642)₃ I JUST COULDN'T THINK ABOUT ANYTHING THAT THAT COULD GET MY MIND OFF OF IT

FIG. 9 (*Loeb*).

A. Occurrences of "Off" or "Out" with S2

	Subject of Clause	Locative
1.	This (Phenobarb)	x
2.	He (Billy)	x
3.	She (Friend II)	x
4.	She (Friend II)	x
5.	that (anything)	x

B. Occurrences of "Off" or "Out" without S2

6.	I		
7.	I	x	
8.	I	x	
9.	I	x	
10.	You're (I)	x	
11.	I	x	
12.	I		
13.	I	x	
14.	I		
15.	I		
16.	I	x	
17.	I		
18.	I		
19.	it		
20.	I		
21.	I		
22.	I	x	
23.	(I)	x	
24.	I		

FIG. 10 (*Loeb*).

her therapy session," which might well include a substrate of "anger," as it might also be present in the single instance of a fear that she might have killed her son. Loeb clearly shows that an individual can use a nonlexical element of expression to reveal ideas to others of which he himself is not conscious. Fourteen of the eighteen fist-like movements described are of less than three seconds duration, and seven of these are less than half of a second in duration. Direct inspection of the film at normal speed reveals that many of these brief fist-like movements could probably *not* be seen with certainty by a psychiatrist in the clinical setting where the film was made even if he deliberately watched the hands of the patient. However, the therapist might well "intuitively" grasp the idea that the patient is angry with him without being able to document those pieces of behavior that evoked his interpretation. Also, it is well known that the psychiatrist might respond in various ways to the patient's anger without ever being conscious himself that he is doing so.[18]

Before embarking on a new series of interactions involving patients, I would like to mention that Condon and Sarles have found splendid synchrony and dyssynchrony in the films of higher primates made by Professors Harry Harlow and Eugene Sackett of Wisconsin. This suggests that primates also live in structured social-communications systems.

A much more difficult and highly controversial aspect of recording synchrony is the correspondence in pulse rate and rhythm, and in electroencephalographic patterns. It is in this latter area where much more work must be done before one can regard the data as verified. Nevertheless, there seem to be synchronous wave forms which correspond to lexical and body motion behavior with the understanding that this aspect of using E.E.G. is only exploratory.

EXPERIMENTS OF A. KENDON AND J. A. SCHOSSBERGER

Adam Kendon, of Oxford University, utilizing the methods of Condon and Ogston, did a close grained analysis of a sound film (TRDOOG) made by Birdwhistell in a London pub in order to study interactional synchrony. He began with genuine scepticism about this phenomenon, but after much hard work convinced himself that it occurred in this context with remarkable precision.[17] I regret I cannot give a detailed description of "the pub scene," but it illustrates remarkable synchrony in two speakers of different cultures with seven other persons present. This is true for a speaker and the person he is addressing, but also as far as can be observed in this sound film, between the speaker and those others present that Kendon calls the "non-axial participants." The precision of this synchrony suggests that all participants, i.e., speakers and listeners, are responding to a rhythm

18 OCCURRENCES OF FISTS
(RIGHT OR LEFT HAND)

Frame Numbers	Anger Words	Statements of Frustration	Statements Denying Anger
(520- 535)₂		X	
(478- 482)₂		X	
(422- 427)₂	X		
(412- 415)₂	X		
(1467- 1468)₁	X		
(1460- 1461)₁	X		
(1459- 1465)₁	X		
(1139-)₁		X	
(1051- 1069)₁			X
(801- 802)₁		X	
(515- 521)₁		X	
(515- 516)₁		X	
(480- 498)₁		X	
(472- 505)₁		X	
(325- 326)₁	X		
(313- 319)₁	X		
(200- 201)₁		X	
(170- 176)₁		X	
Contexts of Fists			

FIG. 11 (*Loeb*).

with which they are thoroughly familiar. As we remarked earlier in the experiment by Sarles, we are highly "programmed" to the rhythm of our speech, and the regular character of the syllabic pulse. Sentences, in terms of stress and intonation patterns and pauses, are highly predictable for the users of a given language. The minute synchrony found by Kendon seems to him to be plausible as a product of the attention of the participants to an input which is highly familiar to them.

Fist	"x" NR	MEN				ANGER-FRUSTRATION						FOOD	NOT MEN		WOMEN	
		Larry	Dr. X	Father	Billy	Anger	Fear	Frustration	Feel	Say, Talk Call	Room House Gate	Eat Food	Not Larry Father Dr. X	Not Billy	Friend II	Friend I
0	NR															
1. (170)1	NR	x														
2. (201)1	NR	x	x		x					x						
3. (313)1	NR				x	x		x								
4. (472)1	NR		x	x				x								
5. (801)1	NR	x						x		x						
6. (1051)1					x	x										
7. (1139)1	NR								x							
8. (1459)1	NR				x	x	x	x								
9. (413)2	NR	x		x	x	x		x	x							
10. (479)2	NR							x								
11. (520)2	NR	x						x		x	x	x				
Foot Back & Forth																
1. (576)1	NR									x						
2. (1136)1	NR															
3. (1305)1	NR									x			x		x	
4. (1331)1	NR											x				
5. (1378)1	NR															
6. (1495)1																x
7. (0001)2											x					x
8. (0025)2	NR															x
9. (0080)2	NR												x			
10. (0109)2	NR												x			
11. (0279)2	NR						x						x			
12. (0290)2	NR												x			
13. (0365)2	NR												x			
14. (0483)2	NR															
15. (0491)2	NR															
16. (0635)2	NR															
17. (0760)2	NR			x												
18. (0783)2	NR													x		
19. (1105)2	NR															
20. (1115)2	NR															
21. (1270)2	NR															
22. (1279)2	NR															
23. (1350)2	NR								x							
24. (0393)3													x			
25. (0389)3													x			
26. (0363)3	NR															

Loeb Dec. 62

FIG. 12 (*Loeb*).

Another experimenter, from a different culture, Dr. J. A. Schossberger of Jerusalem, has also been impressed with the possibilities of close grained studies of sound film. He studied the motility of a little girl, now three and one half years old, who was diagnosed as an autistic child.[29] She had also been diagnosed temporarily as deaf because she did not readily respond to verbal signals, but it was later demonstrated in the film that she does respond to music and other extraneous noises. This shows up well in the sound film. She shows complete synchrony on two occasions with intruding inanimate noncommunicative noise, such as the crackling of a paper bag, and two examples of "postural crumpling" in synchrony with the noise of tapping and a fall of wooden objects on her table.

Schossberger emphasizes the observation made by Condon and others that "observer fatigue" is common and often difficult to overcome when one already knows what is happening on the film. In some instances, many of us have felt revulsion against discovering how strictly determined behavior can be. The discoverer's curiosity must overcome his distaste for what he is looking at, and many who have tried find this too difficult. Schossberger points out that this phenomenon is familiar in psychoanalytic research.

One of the more fascinating observations of Schossberger from the sound film of this little girl is that subsystems may engage in independent synchrony which disrupt the major ongoing movement flow. The synchronous subsystems movement have regularities of their own, can be seen recurrently in appropriate settings and are objective evidence of conflict. In this case the stimulus for these interfering clusters are inanimate sources of intruding noise. Schossberger has high hopes that a true experimental approach to such human relations as identifications, projections and resistance may be made through a close study of the dynamics of the dyadic signal systems.

EXPERIMENTS OF WILLIAM S. CONDON AND WILLIAM OGSTON

It has required several years for Dr. Condon to specify more concretely and in increasing detail the nature of the "unit" of organized behavior as component elements and their regularities were discerned and identified. It is much easier to see them in film than to characterize them verbally, and I will only offer a brief summary from an extensive description. After a futile search for units centered about body parts, Condon found units essentially consisting of an *order* within "a continually changing process." Eyes, arms, legs, etc., *as such*, do not provide the basis for unit status. A "process unit" has stability in the order in which the component elements change together. It is *not* the individual movements taken separately, but the "change-form" of these movements which provides structure, according to Condon. This isomorphism of change of speech and body motion within the speaker is known as self-synchrony.

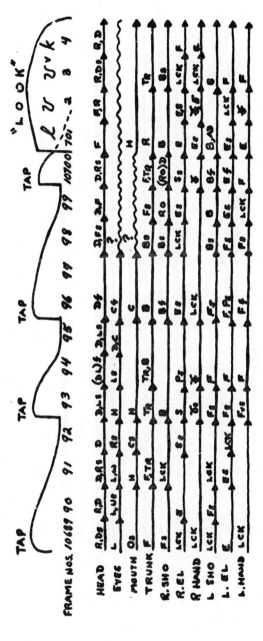

Fig. 13 (*Condon*).—Autistic girl (3½). Marked synchrony with inanimate sound—therapist tapping on object.

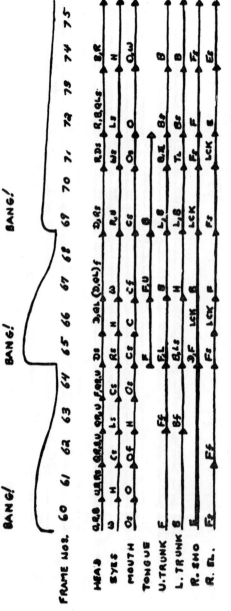

FIG. 14 (*Condon*).—Autistic girl (3½). Marked synchrony with inanimate sound—mother drops blocks.

The "sustaining-and-change" pattern in response to another person is called interactional-synchrony. It is impressive that both have been found to occur consistently over long intervals of film (30 to 60 minutes each) in over fifty films of normal interactants when examined frame by frame. Some of these films were crosscultural, including one of African tribesmen known as the "Kung" who live in the Kahlihari Desert. They have a language based on five clicks, totally unlike ours, yet they can say all they need to and within the framework of the synchronies mentioned.

In view of these demonstrated regularities of both self-synchrony and interactional-synchrony we can now turn to other examples of speech and body motion behavior in patients with (1) aphasia, (2) stuttering, (3)

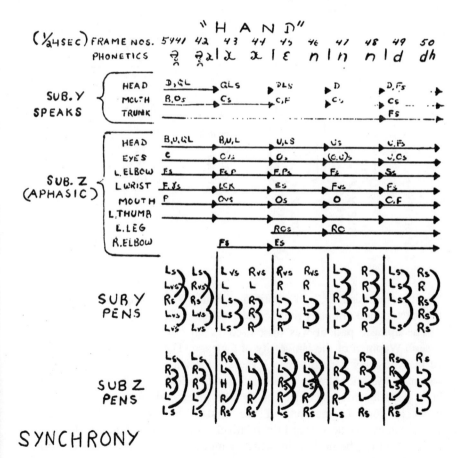

FIG. 15 (Condon).

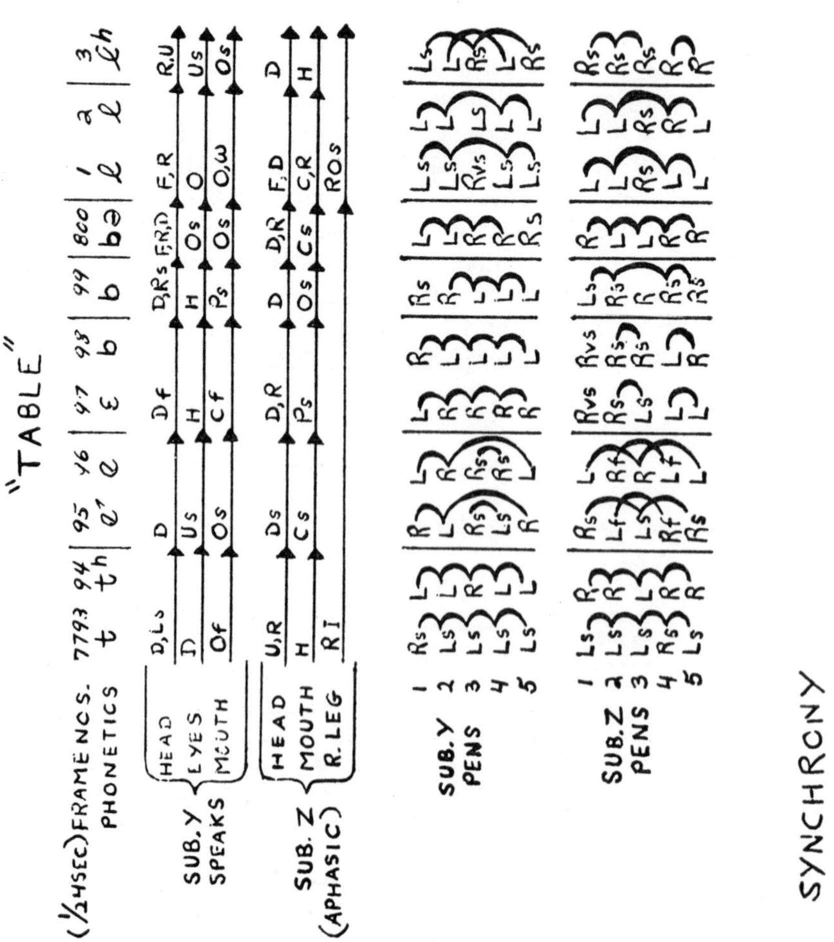

Fig. 16 (*Condon*).

"multiple personality," (4) petit mal, and (5) schizophrenia (three patients examined minutely plus fourteen others which were scanned).

The aphasic patient was diagnosed as an "expressive aphasic" by Dr. Joseph Wepman of the University of Chicago. The sound film shows him to be in synchrony with his speech therapist when she spoke to him, but he becomes dyssynchronous when he tries to speak. In dyssynchrony some body parts are moving out of phase with other body parts, which does not occur in normal synchrony. These figures show clearly that there are numerous events occurring in a relatively brief period. Some of these motions would not be noticed in detail by an observer as they occur at normal speed.

The film of a stuttering patient with his speech therapist shows dyssynchrony at the time of stutter only. His dyssynchrony is similar in form to that of the aphasic patient, but much milder. In Figure 19 he pronounces "ecology" correctly and he is synchronous. The extreme rapidity of individual events is also evident in these figures.

The film of the woman with "multiple personality" known as "The Three Faces of Eve" shows that Eve White had mild dyssynchrony while Eve Black had marked dyssynchrony and marked strabismus. Eve Black had one eye focused on the camera and that side of the face was frowning (asymmetry), while the other eye was focused on the psychiatrist, and that side was smiling. This position was held for several seconds, and then her eyes would move in strange relationship to each other. Jane, the relatively

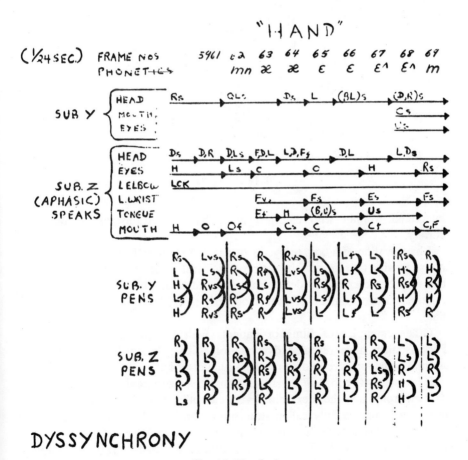

FIG. 17 (Condon).

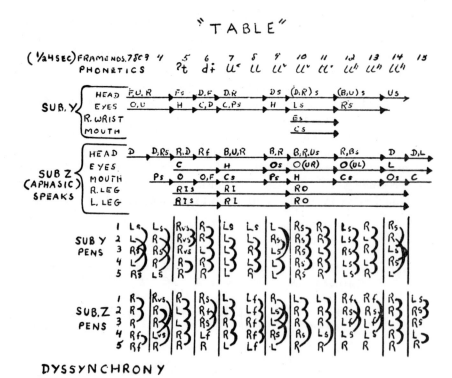

FIG. 18 (*Condon*).

integrated woman who emerged later, had *no* strabismus or dyssynchrony.

I have a slide of a boy, ten years of age, who suffers from petit mal. It is not surprising that he exhibits petit mal, but it may be of interest to see how this may be described in detail from a sound film. This film also shows a relatively large number of events occurring rapidly in a brief period of time.

Other examples of films of patients with Huntington's Chorea and Parkinsonism have revealed dyssynchronies of some order. No films of normal behavior have to date revealed such disorders.

It is noteworthy that *all* seventeen films of schizophrenic patients showed dyssynchrony, and those examined very carefully showed some disorders of eye movements, usually called strabismus, meaning that the eyes did not focus together. Figure 23 shows synchrony between the stutterer and his therapist as he says I.I.T. (Illinois Institute of Technology). The therapist blinks synchronously with his articulation. This is presented to show con-

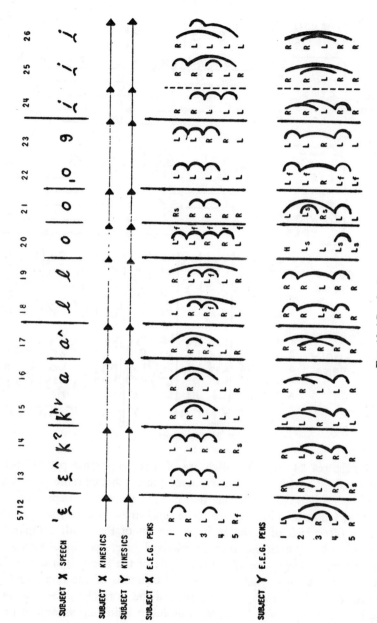

Fig. 19 (*Condon*).

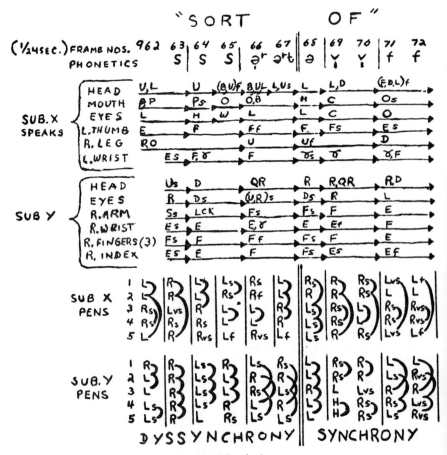

Fig. 20 (*Condon*).

trast with figures 24 and 25, which are of a schizophrenic patient. Space does not permit a detailed description of these schizophrenic patients, a description complicated by the fact that most of them were depressed. The outstanding features, however, are those familiar to you in your practice. There was often lack of variation in movement of the head, comparative rigidity of the head, neck and trunk, prolonged gaze, occasional movement of a body part as if separated from the whole of the body. It is worthwhile to note that the self-dyssynchronies, semi-frozenness of the body, and the "lifelessness" of the speech, changes toward the normal as the patient is said to be better, and may therefore be useful in follow-up as well in prognostic studies.

Among the more interesting findings are the properties of that type of speech characterized by clinicians as "flattened affect". It is described more precisely by Condon, and can be seen on an oscilloscope.[7]

1. There is a smaller than normal range of variation in the degree to which pitch, stress and length vary with each other, and with themselves, from moment to moment.

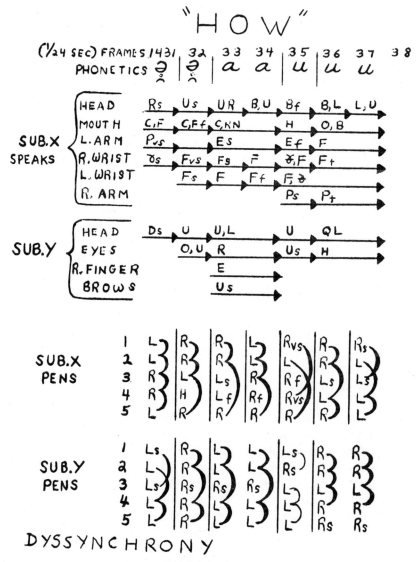

FIG. 21 (Condon).

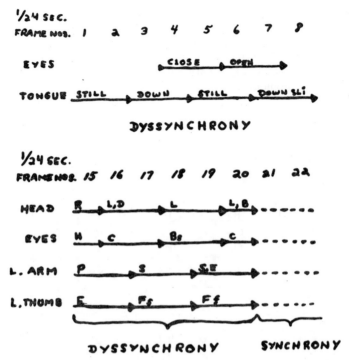

FIG. 22 (*Condon*).—Dissynchrony in boy (10) with petit mal seizure.

2. There is a lack of voice quality or timbre, which is associated with the relative intensity of overtones, or resonance.

3. The terminal contours tend to be relatively level in the sense of lacking the degree of differential slope contained in normal speech.

4. Utterances within the speech stream are broken into segments with pauses between them.

It is noteworthy that, after Condon described these properties, the articles by Stanley S. Newman were called to his attention. In 1939, Newman described these characteristics for depressive reactions, including depressed schizophrenics. Some linguists believe that "flatness" is a more complex phenomenon associated with total appearance and behavior, including reduced motility, eye position, fixed gaze and similar components, but this must be decided by more experimental trials. Perhaps the constriction of pitch and stress are *not* sufficient criteria on linguistic grounds alone. Perhaps those criteria described are appropriate to depressive reactions without being distinctive for schizophrenic reactions without further refinement.[20,21]

The figures of Patient 7, who is schizophrenic, are of interest in that minimal, very rapid dyssynchrony is detectable on sound film when it might escape notice of even a seasoned clinician. In the first figure, the patient is shown while saying, "I admitted into the hospital," in a period slightly longer than one and one-half seconds. There are dyssynchronic changes at almost every frame, with massing of the arrows at major speech points.

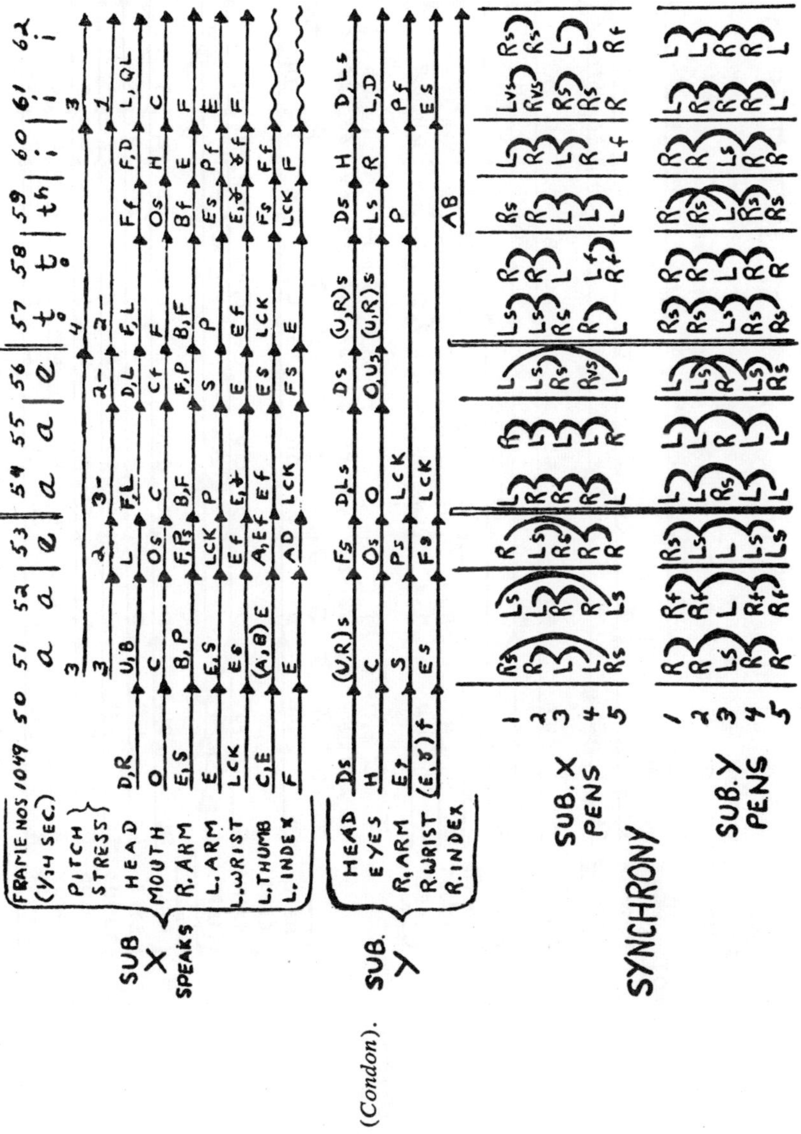

Fig. 23 (*Condon*).

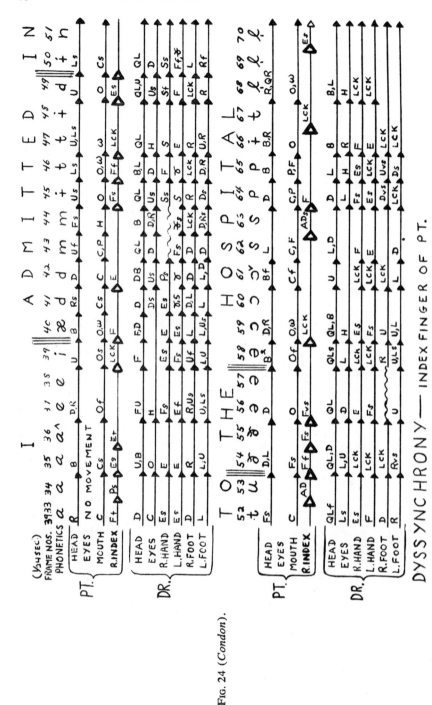

Fig. 24 (*Condon*).

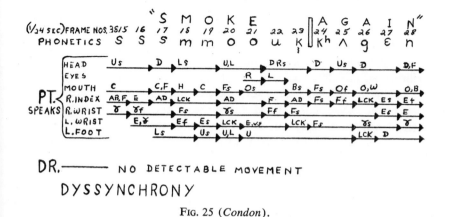

FIG. 25 (*Condon*).

However, both synchrony and dyssynchrony are present, because the patient's head moves in rhythm with his speech while his right index finger moves out of phase and is markedly dyssynchronous. The physician-interviewer moves in synchrony with the head and the speech of the patient.

This dyssynchrony differs in form from that of the other patients such as the aphasic and the stutterer. This schizophrenic patient speaks well, is coherent and relevant, and has an excellent vocabulary. There is no detectable change in the patient's eyes as he stares past the physician. The pitch and stress patterns are severely constricted in contrast to normal speech. His semi-frozen body motion is present throughout the film and, together with his speech, gives a sense of "deadness" to his behavior.

The second figure of Patient 7 shows him saying, "smoke again," in a little over one-half second. Again there are changes at every frame of one-twenty-fourth of a second. Notable is the very rapid and dyssynchronous eye shift toward the camera and back. His speech is not dyssynchronous over a major portion of the two words shown, but there is a hint from additional material that he may become slightly dyssynchronous at areas with "loaded" emotions.

A review of a ten minute film of this interview reveals that both the patient and the doctor are relatively "frozen" compared to normal people. In short periods, there is no detectable change in the body of the doctor. To sustain such lack of change is rare. This leads one to suspect that perhaps the patient's immobile behavior has possibly elicited a reciprocal lack of movement in the doctor's behavior. This could be checked, of course, by viewing his movements with other patients.

It is our hope that after a number of significant patterns have been identified by painstaking search, that they can be much more easily found in successive projects. It also seems likely that they can be put on a computer. I have not discussed the possible correlations with findings from an oscilloscope, but this, too, may be of value. The possibility always exists that better recording at some level of micro or semi-micro will permit a much better study of the therapeutic process and allied interactions. Our material is not yet ready for more than a preliminary public presentation, but my hope is that we can augment current insights considerably by such close-grained analysis.

REFERENCES

1. Bernfeld, S.: Freud's scientific beginnings. *Amer. Imago,* 6:163-196, September, 1949.
2. Bernfeld, S.: Sigmund Freud, M.D., 1882-1885. *Int. J. Psychoanal.* 32:204-217, July, 1951.
3. Braatøy, T. F.: *Fundamentals of Psychoanalytic Technique.* New York, Wiley, 1954.
4. Brosin, H. W.: Linguistic-kinesic analysis using film and tape in a clinical setting. *Amer. J. Psychiat.* 122 (Suppl.): 33-37, June, 1966.
5. Brosin, H. W.: Studies in human communication in clinical settings using sound film and tape. *Wisconsin Med. J.* 63:503-506, November, 1964.
6. Charny, E. J.: Psychosomatic manifestations of rapport in psychotherapy. *Psychosom. Med.* 28: 305-315, July, 1966.
7. Condon, W. S.: *Research Progress Note.* Western Psychiatric Institute and Clinic, September 1, 1967. (Unpublished Manuscript.)
8. Deutsch, F.: Analytic posturology. *Psychoanal. Quart.* 21:196-214, 1952.
9. Deutsch, F.: Correlations of verbal and nonverbal communication in interviews elicited by the associative anamnesis. *Psychosom. Med.* 21:123-130, 1959.
10. Erikson, E. H.: The first psychoanalyst. *Yale Rev.* 46:40-62, 1956.
11. Freud, S.: *A Psycho-Analytic Dialogue: The Letters of Sigmund Freud and Karl Abraham, 1907-1926.* New York, Basic Books, 1965. (See letters following July 6, 1925, p. 382.)
12. Freud, S.: *An Analysis of a Case of Hysteria* (Fragment) (1905). Standard Edition, Vol. 7. London, Hogarth, 1953, pp. 15-122.
13. Freud, S.: *The Question of Lay Analysis* (Postscript) (1927). Standard Edition. Vol. 20. London, Hogarth, 1959, pp. 251-258.
14. Freud, S.: *The Unconscious* (1915). Standard Edition, Vol. 14. London, Hogarth, 1957, pp. 166-204.
15. Gleason, H. A.: *An Introduction to Descriptive Linguistics* (Rev. Ed.). New York, Holt, Rinehart, and Winston, 1961, pp. 2-3.
16. Gottschalk, L. A., and Auerbach, A. H. (Ed.): *Methods of Research in Psychotherapy.* New York, Appleton-Century-Crofts, 1966.
17. Kendon, A.: *Some Observations on Interactional Synchrony.* Pittsburgh, August, 1967. (Unpublished Manuscript.)
18. Loeb, F. F.: *The Fist.* Pittsburgh, 1967. (Unpublished Manuscript.)

19. Meyer, A.: British influences in psychiatry and mental hygiene: The fourteenth Maudsley lecture: *J. Ment. Sci.* 79: 435-63, 1933. Also *in* Meyer, A.: *The Collected Papers of Adolf Meyer* (E. E. Winters, Gen. Ed.). Baltimore, Johns Hopkins Press, 1950-52, Vol. 3, pp. 400-428.

20. Newman, S. S., and Mather, V. G.: Analysis of spoken language of patients with affective disorders. *Amer. J. Psychiat.* 94:913-942, 1938.

21. Newman, S. S.: Personal symbolism in language patterns. *Psychiatry* 2:177-184, 1939.

22. Pike, K. L.: *Language in Relation to a Unified Theory of the Structure of Human Behavior.* The Hague, Mouton, 1967.

23. Pike, K. L.: Towards a theory of the structure of human behavior. *Gen. Syst.* 2:135-141, 1957.

24. Ritvo, L. B.: *Darwin of the Mind: The Influence of Darwin on Freud as Revealed in the 19th Century Life and Works of Freud.* New Haven, Yale University, 1963. (Unpublished Dissertation.)

25. Sapir, E.: *Selected Writings in Language, Culture and Personality* (D. G. Mandelbaum, Ed.). Berkeley, University of California Press, 1949.

26. Scheflen, A. E. *Behavioral Programs in Human Communication.* 1967. (Unpublished Manuscript.)

27. Scheflen, A. E.: *Strategy and Structure in Psychotherapy.* Philadelphia, Eastern Pennsylvania Psychiatric Institute, 1965.

28. Scheflen, A. E.: *Stream and Structure of Communicational Behavior: Context Analysis of a Psychotherapy Session.* Philadelphia, Eastern Pennsylvania Psychiatric Institute, 1965.

29. Schossberger, J. A.: *People and Things, Kinesic Synchrony, and Intentional Schisis in One Case of Infantile Autism.* Pittsburgh, 1967. (Unpublished Manuscript.)

30. *Symposium on Expression of the Emotions in Man,* New York, 1960. Held at American Association for the Advancement of Science Meeting, December 29-30, 1960 (P. H. Knapp, Ed.). New York, International Universities Press, 1963.

31. *Webster's Seventh New Collegiate Dictionary.* Springfield, Mass., G. & C. Merriam Company, 1963.

Biological Research Developments in Psychiatry

FRANCIS J. BRACELAND, M.D.

"Man can do a great deal by observation and thinking, but with them alone he cannot unravel the mysteries of Nature. Had it been possible, the Greeks would have done it; and could Plato and Aristotle have grasped the value of experiment in the progress of human knowledge, the course of European history might have been very different."

Alan Gregg*

IT DOES SEEM somewhat presumptuous for a clinician lately turned editor to try to assess the impact of biological research developments upon the discipline of psychiatry. It is an overwhelming task! There is much too much activity and too much overlap to do the subject justice in a short presentation of this type. Technical advances are forcing reevaluation of many of the developments we once thought settled. Still, withal, our knowledge is deficient and the etiologies of the most important disorders still elude our grasp.

In most of the meetings of basic scientists, the clinician humbly acknowledges his debt to their efforts and knows that without their help his discipline would be off in the ineffectual reaches of capricious imagination. I now make this acknowledgement here again. Sadly, at times, we seek to understand the various brilliant new scientific findings and the potentials they hold for the future, and are forced to conclude that clinicians and basic scientists often seem to inhabit different worlds.

I will approach the problem assigned to me from a somewhat different angle and note that while we have advanced in our basic studies in incredible fashion, the same problems concern us which concerned our medical ancestors: namely, what is psychiatry's place in medicine and what is medicine's place among the sciences? Conversely, this would mean what is the impact of the biological sciences upon medicine, upon psychiatry, and upon the clinician? Both Sir Francis Walshe[23] in his Harveian oration in 1948, and Alan Gregg[11] in his Terry Lectures at Yale in 1941, addressed

---

*Quoting Theobald Smith, *American Journal of Medical Science,* December 1929, p. 24.[11]

themselves to some of the same questions we seek to answer here and it is probable that I would do well simply to quote these estimable gentlemen and in that way place myself safe from criticism, under the protection of their intellectual umbrellas. However, neither you nor they would approve of that.

Both men were painfully aware, as am I, of the essentiality of basic research, and aware, also, of the fact that it cannot be the be all and end all of medical practice. As Gregg noted:

> It is not infrequently taken for granted that the results of laboratory research are final and its operations infallible. This however is far from true. The laws, theories, and inferences of experimental research are as subject to rectification as are inferences based on other human activities. They are approximations getting nearer and nearer the actuality with time.

Walshe approached the same problem in another fashion:

> Whether a scientific process or method can be applied, science when introduced into medicine depends upon the rational basis of its use. It is therefore salutary to remind ourselves that the fruits of scientific discovery irrationally employed do not constitute applied science in medicine. Indeed, the practical arts in diagnosis, prognosis, and treatment continue to take a prominent and essential place in our activities. They may be relatively inexact and have no ascertained scientific basis, yet they embody the sagacity of our predecessors, and they demand in those who employ them an aptitude and an intuition that many modern procedures of more pretentious and scientific pedigree do not always require, and often do not obtain, from those who use them with a suave assurance of being highly scientific.

The necessity of our taking a connected view of the old and the new, the past and the present, the science and the art if we are to be skilled clinicians is thus apparent. As we find ourselves in the process of trying to build a foundation for a more complete understanding of man, we look not only to the basic physical and biological sciences for help, but also to every branch of the sciences and humanities that touch upon our clinical practice. By adapting and modifying their methods and procedures, we can devise procedures of our own to help us find some explanation of how complex systems are associated with normal and abnormal behavior. Applied to the problems of psychiatry, the valuable findings of these sciences can render our approach to the care of the mentally ill more scientific and more effective.

Viewed in a larger context, some of the theories and developments in the biological sciences that seem valid and exciting to us now may prove questionable and impractical later on; but hypotheses that cannot be substantiated now may eventually provide just the clues we seek to the etiology of mental disorders and thus even delineate the guidelines for prevention. According to Henry David Thoreau:

No way of thinking or doing, however ancient, can be trusted without proof. What everybody echoes or in silence passes by as true today may turn out to be falsehood tomorrow, mere smoke of opinion.[21]

Thus, now that you are thoroughly and somewhat lugubriously warned, we can take a brief overview of some of the biological research in progress in various fields today and see perchance if they have potentialities for helping us understand the problems which face us. Necessarily, this overview must be limited and highly selective.

GENETICS

As in the Scriptures, the place to begin is in the beginning. Therefore, we should first consider genetics, for its students seek fundamental causes of personality deviations. It is hard to believe that 90 per cent of the detailed information available on human genetics was not known ten years ago.

The late Franz Kallmann, who was one of the moving spirits in this highly active research field, noted that it is no longer possible to relegate human heredity to the status of a mysterious force and that we now have sufficiently penetrating techniques for tracing psychopathological conditions, theoretical deduction and impersonal extrapolation. Through concerted action, they form a science of genetics *applied to people,* to benefit people, and to be understood by people for their own good and that of their progeny. This statement fits in very well with our present thesis.

Dr. John D. Rainer, a colleague of the late Kallman's, has pointed out that genetic concepts can be incorporated into clinical management in a psychotherapeutic setting, can be effective in the areas of child psychiatry and advice on child rearing, and, in general, in the keener understanding of a patient within his family constellation. He said:

> Working at the molecular, chemical, physiological, psychological, and demographic levels, and welding together psychodynamic and physiodynamic considerations, genetics can become the finest vehicle for an integrated approach to psychopathology.[16]

For a while, the hopes we had for one aspect of this vehicle, namely, that DNA would prove to be a carrier of species information and RNA a carrier of day to day information, and thus simplify the general concept of transfer of information in biochemical form from one animal to another, seemed to be dashed. But now converts seem to be coming over to that thesis. Ungar, of Baylor University,[22] in a more modest claim, says only that partial purification of some of the transfer factors of learned behavior showed them to be peptides or proteins. Ersman and Lehrer,[7] reporting in the same volume, suggest that RNA extracts from the brains of donor mice trained to a specific task, facilitate learning in that task by naive animals.

Perhaps at this time we are safe in assuming modestly that some lines of recent study afford strong evidence that RNA may, indeed, constitute the substance for storage of day-to-day information. The potentialities of this type of research are obviously of great interest to the psychiatrist.

There have been a number of basic twin studies beginning with the work of Luxenburger in 1928 and including the classical studies of Kallman and Slater. For the most part, they indicated that adult schizophrenic concordance percentages were between 58 per cent and 69 per cent for monozygotic twins in contrast to 0 to 17 per cent for dizygotic twins of the same sex. However, later studies find less concordance in schizophrenia for the monozygotic twins, namely, 42 per cent concordance for them versus 9 per cent for dizygotic twins of the same sex.[10] In this regard, Gottesman, in a recent report, concluded that the mode of transmission of schizophrenia was quite complex and suggested a polygenic theory with or without a major gene.

A note in one of the medical news journals published July 13, 1967, reporting on the Conference on the Transmission of Schizophrenia held in Puerto Rico, stated that Heston, of the University of Iowa, reported that a detailed study of forty-seven persons born to schizophrenic mothers, but separated permanently from them and from maternal relatives shortly after birth, gave fresh support to a genetic origin of schizophrenia. He stated that:

> The study of these experimental subjects and fifty matched controls also yielded another totally unexpected finding; it produced no evidence that institutional care during childhood had any effect on adult psychosocial adjustment. Schizophrenia was found in 5 of the 47 offspring of schizophrenic mothers and in none of the control group.

It is obvious that the report on institutional care differs markedly from our usual thinking in this regard.

Still another report from that same conference[2] dealt with adopted children and Kety, et al., examined the records of 5500 such children in a three-phase research project. To brief their report, perhaps to the point of oversimplification, we note that the researchers believed they had proof that heredity plays an important role in schizophrenia. However they add, "It is not schizophrenia which is inherited. Rather, the genes may lead to a variety of abnormalities."

Further evidence of this fact was added by Pollin and Stabenau[2] at the same meeting. They reported on a situation in which one twin was normal and one was schizophrenic. They concluded that:

> Nongenetic biological factors from the child's prenatal life played a part in initiating a whole sequence of events relating to the presence or absence of the

disease. (These factors were such things as position of the unborn, weight, susceptibility to infection of the infant, etc.).

Thus, adding up the factors adduced thus far in the various researches, we may surmise that while genetic control of schizophrenia is unlikely, direct attack upon underlying metabolic and other factors is likely to be fruitful.

PSYCHOPHYSIOLOGY

The relatively new specialty of psychophysiology, concerned with the study of behavior and its underlying psychological and physiological correlates, is seen to hold great promise for practical applications in our clinical practice. Electrocardiography, electroencephalography, blood pressure, gastrointestinal mobility, body temperature, bodily activity and blood chemistry, all have been simultaneously observed and correlated with normal and abnormal behavior in living and fully conscious animals—a remarkable step forward—made possible by technological advances and instruments which only lately have appeared on the scene.

It is the hope of this young science that, in addition to overt behavioral deviations, covert physiologic deviations might be found which would assist in categorizing, understanding and treating the various kinds of mental illness. However, despite the biologic implications of widespread psychiatric use of psychoactive drugs, the search for clinical physiologic correlates of disturbed behavior has not been overly successful. Last year, however, detailed longitudinal studies of neurosis formation revealed that certain physiological mechanisms utilized in the onset and development of disturbed behavior are apparently not necessary for sustaining such behavior. This evidence gives us greater insight into this enigma and eventually parallels in human behavior may be revealed.

By analogy, careful hospital study of a disturbed patient usually does not occur for some weeks, months or years after the onset and developmental stages of the illness; etiologic correlations of a physiologic nature, which initially might have been clearly evident, have conceivably undergone adaptation and are no longer apparent. Persistent and subtle biochemical variations may yet be detected, although the problems of sampling such changes against the context of adaptation of the whole organism is certainly a formidable task.

Awareness of the dilemma this poses could understandably lead many investigators to a pessimistic point of view, but it is in projects such as this that the methods of the experimental scientist could be serviceable to the clinical investigator and practitioner.

The research strategy of making many measurements on an individual subject over a long period of time has begun to yield unexpected, even startling, results. When the physiologic functioning of subjects is measured many times each day over a period of weeks, we find very consistent twenty-four hour changes dependent not on eating or sleeping times but on internal "biologic clocks," as ably described by Dr. Curt P. Richter in his *Biologic Clocks in Medicine and Psychiatry*. Other workers have suggested that these clocks play an important role in regulating the homeostatic mechanisms of the many organs in the body. On the basis of preliminary data, it has been reported that one pervasive correlate of disturbed behavior in monkeys is a deterioration of the ability of these clocks to keep accurate time. They tend to go slower or lose time as behavior becomes increasingly disturbed. However, when the administration of certain psychoactive drugs is successful in reducing the disturbed behavior, a simultaneous improvement has been observed in the time being kept by a monkey's inner clock. Of course, no statement can yet be made about cause and effect relationships in this association of disturbed behavior, drugs and biologic clocks as physiologic correlates. Nonetheless, the possibilities that suggest themselves for human trials based on similar methods stir the imagination. Perhaps they may even indicate optimal times of day for the dosage of drugs. At present, efforts are being made in our own laboratories under Dr. Stroebel[20] to determine this, as the physiological and behavioral reactions of laboratory animals are being monitored by computer, twenty-four hours a day, seven days a week.

Before touching upon pharmacological discoveries which have meant so much to the clinician, we might take a moment to note that the general hospitals' medical and surgical wards offer an exciting hunting ground for the basic scientist. There the clinician is faced with many questions which as yet have not been answered for him. Why is it that the psychiatrist is often first to see the individual who is depressed, has lost weight, has abdominal pain and an intractible insomnia plus a feeling of impending disaster, and who many times turns out to have carcinoma of the pancreas? Why the emotional accompaniments of low blood sugar, unrest, neurosis, manic attacks and alcoholism? Why do many patients operated upon for adrenal pathology become paranoid? These are but a few of the problems which face the clinician and prove to him that one's psyche and soma can never be considered as separate and discrete entities.

PHARMACOLOGY

It is not my intention to discuss either pharmacology or psychopharmacology in detail. You are as well informed as am I about both disciplines. Pharmacology established a place in psychiatry over a decade ago and produced major excitement as the so-called phenotropic drugs appeared upon the scene. While they have helped immeasurably to relieve agitation and depression in many individuals, particularly those hospitalized, we still do not understand exactly how they work and we still have a great deal to learn about the effects of individual drugs under a variety of conditions. Some of the preparations which aroused great interest ten years ago are still under careful study and one has the feeling that things are falling slowly into place and that we are now ready, as a result of technological advances and invention of new apparatus, to study their modes of action in a much more sophisticated manner.

No new drugs of the calibre of chlorpromazine, imipramine or the MAO inhibitors have appeared on the scene of late, but at present there is marked interest in combinations of drugs already approved and in use. Wide acceptance is reported of the clinical usefulness of combinations of perphenazine and amitriptyline. This tends to substantiate what previously was a hunch concerning the synergistic actions of other combinations such as trifluoperazine and tranylcypromine, dextro amphetamine and amylbarbital, etc., and all of this may presage a new psychopharmacologic development.

AFFECTIVE DISORDERS

Although some investigators have called his thesis into question, Schildkraut, in his excellent paper, *The Catecholamine Hypothesis of Affective Disorder. A Review of Supporting Evidence*,[18] concluded that:

> The Catecholamine hypothesis of affective disorders proposes that some, if not all, depressions are associated with an absolute or relative decrease in catecholamines, particularly norepinephrine available at central adrenergic receptor sites. Elation, conversely, may be associated with an excess of such amines.

It was this hypothesis that he reviewed and, although he could neither affirm nor reject it on the basis of available data, nevertheless said:

> In our present state of knowledge, the hypothesis is of considerable heuristic value, providing the investigator and the clinician with a frame of reference integrating much of our experience with those pharmacological agents which produce alterations in human affective states.

The value of this research to the clinician is important mostly for what it promises for the future. (Incidentally, Schildkraut's paper, *Norepinephrine Metabolism and Psychoactive Drugs in Depression*, was recently awarded the much sought after German Dortmund prize of $10,000 in competition with researchers from all over the world.)

Thus as we get closer to an understanding of the underlying biochemistry of depressions which Kraines and many others have insisted are biological disorders, clinicians find themselves in difficulty because they have trouble defining and differentiating these illnesses which are as old as man's recorded history. Interestingly enough, it has taken the differences of opinion regarding imipramine and electric shock to point up our difficulties even more sharply.

It was noted in a recent World Congress that Americans are using different categories and a somewhat different nomenclature to describe depressions than our European colleagues, and differences of this kind obviously will interfere with proper scientific reporting. Fortunately, the NIMH has decided to convene a small group of scientists to attempt to bring order out of this nosologic chaos. At present the understanding and categorization of depression is a shambles. Though the diagnosis is the one most frequently made in psychiatry today, it covers everything from a mild attack of "the blues" to malignant suicidal depressive episodes.

The use of lithium carbonate in the treatment of manic depressive patients, manic type, should be mentioned briefly. It has been found in a number of instances to be extremely effective in controlling manic excitement. Patients have done very well and, in most instances reported, have had no recurrence of either manic or depressive symptoms. It is true that some unfortunate side effects have been reported in the use of the drug, and the F.D.A. has recently seen fit to issue a warning about its use, calling attention to the fact that it is still investigational and has various toxic side effects. However, the consensus among investigators is that the difficulties which do arise in the giving of the drug are most frequently due to improper dosage and to lack of an accompanying administration of sodium. One of the most recent reports[17] of successful and uneventful treatment noted: "At the dosage level used, blood lithium levels approached 0.7 meq/L on the fourth day of treatment. This amount decreased as maintenance dosage was established and serum levels stabilized between 0.5 meq/L and 0.3 meq/L." These blood levels are much lower than those reported by individuals who have had difficulties.

In order to avoid serious toxicity, the authors quoted gave each patient 4 Gm. of sodium chloride daily and had patients omit lithium one day each week and stop taking it during febrile illnesses.

Present day interest in LSD has renewed previously suspended studies on the psychotomimetic effects of mescaline. Unfortunately the final answers to the influence of these drugs have not been written because they have become a cause for partisan quarrel following their injudicious usage in nonmedical settings. Dr. Harold Abramson,[14] one of the most knowledgeable investigators of this drug, having used it over the period of twenty years in some alcoholic patients, is well persuaded of its use, as is Lauretta Bender, who has used it in treatment of autistic children. It is apparent that many clinicians are poorly informed about the drug, for although Abramson notes that more than 1000 scientific papers have been written about it over the past two decades, to many of us that fact is new.

It is noteworthy in this regard that Ruth Fox[8] reported that, in addition to LSD, sixteen of twenty severe recalcitrant alcoholics showed improvement *with the total push method and few of the patients could say which form of the treatment was of most help to them.* Medical investigators have been careful to keep the dosage of the drug within safe limits and practically all of them decry its use by nonmedical personnel.

Meanwhile, the number of mental hospital admissions with LSD psychoses grows monthly, the victims usually young people and marginal types, and the distressing part of the problem is that psychotic reactions can recur weeks or even months after the initial exposure. At present, research is in progress to determine the proper use of this category of drugs.

Recent reports in the lay press note that researchers at the State University of New York at Buffalo reported LSD caused chromosomes to break in human blood cells grown in a test tube. In pregnant laboratory rats, the drug is said to have a thalidomide-like effect in the offspring. The same research group also indicated that some of the tranquilizing drugs in common use had the same effect. Unfortunately, the reports of these researchers are not yet available for scientific evaluation.

While there is much more basic biologic research going on at present, we can only mention some of it here in passing. The collaborative efforts of Hoagland, Freeman, Berger and Pennell of the Worcester Foundation and Medfield State Hospital are examples in point. They are of the opinion that Heath's taraxin is the same as their fraction PGP. Both produced spiking in electrical recording from electrodes chronically implanted in the septum of monkeys. These disturbances, Hoagland[4] reports, were accompanied in the monkeys by catatonic-like behavior. We will say more about Heath's work later. Before we do, however, a few words should be said about microchemistry and about sleep and dream research.

Microchemists[5] are investigating the chemical properties of very small areas of the central nervous system. Since it has been shown that separate areas of the brain are characterized by different chemical properties, a microchemical study has the potential of defining the chemical basis of various regulatory areas of the brain. There is much more work to be done, however, before this discipline can contribute of its leaven, if that it proves to be.

As to sleep and dreams, since present day research findings are well known, it is unnecessary to dwell deeply upon them. Whether, as Snyder maintains, the REM state is a separate state between sleep and dreaming, or whether it is not, as Dement insists, seems to be a matter of semantics. Snyder conjectures that REM serves a sentinel function—a built-in mechanism which provides maximal security with minimal disturbance of sleep, thus preparing the organism for flight or fight. Initially, it probably aided the survival advantage of the early mammalian predicament. One interesting and hopeful fact, as Snyder observes, is that most of the work done thus far on the REM state has been by psychiatrists and one welcomes that trend.

In an interesting conclusion to a very careful study of the dream, Whitman et al.[24] observe with Kety that, "We may someday have a biochemistry of memory, but not of memories, and this holds true for dreaming and dreams. Though biology and psychology meet in the dream process, each has its own uniqueness."

SCHIZOPHRENIA

Although we are all aware that present thinking regards the biological aspects of schizophrenia as only one part of the problem, and thus far a small one, yet researchers hunt diligently for some biological disorder which might, if understood, bring the illness under control. It is generally believed that both schizophrenia and the manic depressive syndromes are associated with some metabolic disorders. This in no way lessens the importance of psychological factors for it is probable that they modify the development of the underlying biochemical abnormality.

In a recent British symposium, J. R. Smythies[19] noted that various studies had come to make this association because:

1. There is evidence of a generic factor in the illness.
2. There is no actual definite discoverable psychological predisposition in many cases.
3. We now know two conditions, where a condition clinically undistinguishable from paranoid schizophrenia is produced by a physical cause, viz., temporal lobe epilepsy and chronic amphetamine addiction.

There are many suggestive findings of a metabolic substance in schizophrenia, but none is definite as to the etiology of the disorder. We can only mention general directions in this limited survey.

Himwich[13] believes that there are presently two main trends suggesting hypothesis for biochemical abnormalities associated with schizophrenia, and adds a third trend which has to do with depressions.

He notes that the first hypothesis was put forth in 1952 by Osmond, Harley-Mason and Smythies,[15] based on the observation that the hallucinogenic drug mescaline is a close chemical relative of noradrenaline. They suggested that schizophrenia may be associated with a metabolic fault whereby a mescaline-like compound, dimethoxyphenylethylamine might be hallucinogenic and give rise to clinical disorder of schizophrenics. From this viewpoint, schizophrenia is associated with the production in the body of a specific mescaline-like abnormal metabolite.

The next step came in 1962, when Friedhoff and Van Winkle[9] reported an isolated mescaline-like compound dimethoxyphenylethylamine (DMPE) from schizophrenic urine, the so-called pink spot. This viewpoint is still controversial. It seems that certain schizophrenics do excrete this compound which is ordinarily not found in normal urines. At the present time it seems unlikely that the patients form DMPE, and some investigators have allied the pink spot to diet. Another hypothesis was suggested by Brune and Himwich[6] in 1962. They had previously found (1960) that tryptamine appeared in the urine before the patient became worse, remained high in the urine during the period of behavioral worsening and was restored to original values when the patient's behavior improved. Tryptamine is a breakdown product of tryptophan, an essential amino acid.

The second attack on the problem of schizophrenia originated with Himwich and his colleagues.[3] Using the technique originated by Dr. Kety and his group, they gave methionine to schizophrenic patients who were on MAO inhibitor medication, i.e., marplan or parnate. Again they found an increase in tryptamine in the urine with exacerbations of symptoms and postulated at that time that a psychotogenic tryptamine compound was formed with the methyl groups obtained from methionine. Next they uncovered the fact that this substance is formed endogenously in the body and in the last year, by three different methods, proved that bufotenin, a psychotogenic substance, is in the urine together with more strongly psychotogenic ones, but confirmed the latter by only one method. Both hypotheses depend upon a methylation of a substance which would otherwise not be psychotogenic.

Finally, they believe there is an indication that some of the depressions, but not all, are associated with the diminished serotonin content in the brain. There is much evidence that the breakdown product of serotonin is decreased during some of the depressions and Coppen et al. (1964) pointed out that the ability of the brain of some depressed patients to form serotonin from its precursor is impaired, and this is a biochemical correlate in a large group of depressed patients.

You can see from these directions that the whole field of biochemistry is active and it is obvious that one of the first things to be done is to definitely identify the "pink spot" chemically and correlate it with the clinical situation in longitudinal studies.

The studies of Gottlieb and Heath and their colleagues continue. Heath[12] has now been working for nearly twenty years on his postulate that schizophrenia is an immunologic disorder. A gamma immuno globulin

(1gG) fraction of sera of schizophrenic patients has been observed to alter brain function by combining with antigenic sites of neural cell nuclei of the septal region and thereby probably interfering with neurohumoral conductors to produce physiologic changes and behavioral symptoms. This psychosis-inducing 1gG fraction antibody or antibody simulator has been found in sera of acutely psychotic schizophrenic patients in high enough titer to be demonstrable by passive transfer in volunteer nonpsychotic recipients and in rhesus monkeys.

At the 1967 convention of the American Psychiatric Association, Heath noted that:

> We are approaching a definition of a clear cut pathologic entity based on objective biologic findings. But simpler laboratory demonstration with consistent duplication of our findings in other laboratories is required before a clearly biologic definition of schizophrenia will gain wide acceptance.[11]

Heinz Lehman,[14] a careful scientist who discussed Heath's paper at the same meeting, indicated that he had witnessed in a few instances what he thinks were probably true taraxein reactions and found it a fascinating experience. He, too, believes that this problem must be tackled again in one or more laboratories outside of New Orleans. He adds, however, "Even if confirmed, the anti-brain antibody theory of the Tulane group may explain only a certain proportion of acute schizophrenic breakdowns. Nevertheless, today the Taraxein Theory of schizophrenia must be considered one of the most challenging unsolved problems in psychiatric research."

This overview has become more extensive than I had originally intended, even though it merely touches the surface of the biologic research now going on in psychiatry. In closing, I would like to return to Alan Gregg for, with him, I sum up my thoughts on the subject matter I have discussed:

> Great as might be the benefits from a far more extensive support of research in medicine, I do not advocate medical research making promises beyond its powers to redeem. Even after science has given us all she can supply, we shall depend upon the unique rewards of morality and religion to make human existence acceptable to man. How the facts of science are to be applied, for what purposes and to whose benefit, are questions not yet to be settled by science. We cannot sensibly look to medical science for what it cannot provide. Canons of taste, standards of value, a code of morals are not within the sphere of science. It is part of the confusion of the modern mind to look to science for everything that is helpful and willfully to ignore her when she warns, "I can show you how but I cannot tell you why to do things."[11]

This expresses more elegantly how this particular clinician and editor looks at basic studies—a view which has not been particularly popular in this present day and age, but one which I think offers one more step toward the understanding of people suffering with mental disease, and anything which helps in that direction is particularly welcome.

REFERENCES

1. Abramson, H.: *The Uses of LSD in Psychotherapy and Alcoholism.* Indianapolis, Bobbs Merrill, 1966.
2. American Psychiatric Association: Studies link adoptees' heredity prenatal life to schizophrenia. *Psychiat. News,* August 1967, p. 23.
3. Berlet, H. H., Bull, C., Himwich, H. E., Kohl, H., Matsumoto, K., Pscheidt, G. R., Spaide, J., Tourlentes, T. T., and Valverde, J. M.: Endogenous metabolic factor in schizophrenic behavior. *Science* 144:311, 1964.
4. Berger, J. R.: Biologic concomitants of schizophrenia. *Ment. Hyg.* 50(4):507, October 1966.
5. Braceland, F. J.: Applied research. *Ment. Hyg.* 50(4):561, October 1966.
6. Brune, G. G., and Himwich, H. E.: Effects of methionine loading on the behavior of schizophrenic patients. *J. Nerv. Ment. Dis.* 134:447, 1962.
7. Ersman, W. B., and Lehrer, G. H.: Facilitation of maze performance by RNA extracts from maze trained mice. *Fed. Proc.* 1967, 21(2).
8. Fox, R.: A multidisciplinary approach to the treatment of alcoholism. *Amer. J. Psychiat.* 123(7):769-778, January 1967.
9. Friedhoff, A. J., and Van Winkle, E.: Isolation and characterization of a compound from the urine of schizophrenics. *Nature (Lond.)* 194:897, 1962.
10. Gottesman, and Shields: *In* Maher, B. A. (Ed.): *Progress in Experimental Personality Research,* Vol. 3. New York, Academic Press, 1966.
11. Gregg, A.: *The Furtherance of Medical Research (The Terry Lectures).* New Haven, Yale University Press, 1941, p. 7.
12. Heath, R. G., and Krupp, I. M.: Schizophrenia as a specific biologic disease. In press. (Paper delivered at APA Convention, 1967.)
13. Himwich, H.: Personal communication.
14. Lehman, H.: *Discussion of Heath/Krupp Paper* (at APA Convention, 1967).
15. Osmond, H., and Smythies, J. R.: Schizophrenia: A new approach. *J. Ment. Sci.* 98:309, 1952.
16. Rainer, J. D.: Studies in the genetics of disordered behavior: Methods and objectives. Chapter *in* Kallman, F. J. (Ed.): *Expanding Goals of Genetics in Psychiatry.* New York, Grune & Stratton, 1962, p. 3.
17. Schagenhauf, G., Tupin, J., and White, R. B.: The use of lithium carbonate in the treatment of manic psychoses. *Amer. J. Psychiat.* 123(8):201, August 1966.
18. Schildkraut: The catecholamine hypothesis of affective disorder. A review of supporting evidence. *Amer. J. Psychiat.* 122:509-522, November 1965.
19. Smythies, J. R.: Recent advances in the biochemistry of schizophrenia. *In* Coppen, A., and Walk, A. (Eds.): *Recent Developments in Schizophrenia—A Symposium.* (Brit. J. Psychiat., Spec. Publ. #1). Ashford Kent, Headley Bros. for the Royal Medico-Psychological Assoc., 1967, pp. 61-68.
20. Stroebel, C.: Personal communication.
21. Thoreau, H. D.: Walden. *In: Walden and Selected Essays.* Chicago, Packard, 1941, p. 3.
22. Ungar, G.: Transfer of learned information by brain extracts. *Fed. Proc.* 26(2):263, 1967.
23. Walshe, F.: *The Structure of Medicine and Its Place Among the Sciences.* (Harveian Oration, RCP London.) Edinburgh, Livingston, 1948, p. 19.
24. Whitman, R. M., Kramer, M., Ornstein, P. H., and Baldridge, W. J.: The physiology, psychology and utilization of dreams. *Amer. J. Psychiat.* 124(3):287-302, September 1966.

Psychiatric Services in Colleges

DANA L. FARNSWORTH, M.D.

COLLEGE PSYCHIATRY has enjoyed a slow but steady growth since its first applications in higher education. College officials' interest in it has increased at a rapid rate since World War II. But shortage of psychiatrists trained and interested in the field has slowed the development of effective college psychiatric services. Many colleges and universities now recognize the desirability of developing good mental services as part of their total counseling program, but are unable to secure the appointment of a full-time psychiatrist. Some can only obtain the services of a psychiatrist for a few hours each week; in such instances he must of necessity spend most of his time seeing only the acutely disturbed or consulting with those who are in varying degrees responsible for students in emotional conflict.

But is there a special need for psychiatrists on college health services that could not be met by sending those who needed treatment to private practitioners, assuming that such were available in all college communities? Certainly the number of students who became ill enough to require hospitalization for mental disorders would not justify a college psychiatric service, welcome as it may be when acute emergencies occur. Experience over the past decade at the Harvard University Health Services (which is characteristic of most educational institutions with adequate psychiatric coverage), indicates that only about 2 to 3 students per 1,000 enrolled will require removal to a hospital each year.[10; p.6]

Such an estimate in no way reflects the real justification for college psychiatrists. Suicide attempts are frequent in nearly all colleges, there being usually from three to six attempts for every suicide accomplished. Saving the lives or careers of those students who survive the attempt involves not only intensive and prompt care, but also the development of an understanding and awareness of the significance of suicide attempts among all members of the college community. When this occurs the chances of early recognition and making help available in time are greatly increased.

At the Harvard University Health Services, more than 11 per cent of all students seek and receive help each year. Women, medical students and theological students use the services most frequently (15 to 19 per cent yearly), and other graduate students use it least (about 8.5 per cent). Male undergraduates fall in the intermediate range (about 14 per cent). Many factors influence the decision to seek help—availability, attitudes toward psychiatry, confidence in individual psychiatrists, etc.—but it seems unlikely that any single group is basically more prone to emotional disorder than any others. Many students receive psychiatric help privately and are not known to the health services, probably a third as many as come to the health services.

Various combinations of depression and anxiety account for the vast majority of students who seek help. Were psychiatric help not readily available, many of these would consult other sources of help (friends, parents, counselors, ministers or priests), while others would deal with their problems unaided. Some would not even be aware that it is proper to seek help in conflict resolution. Critics of college psychiatry say that the awareness of need for psychiatric help should not be encouraged, but if this is not done the serious problems usually must be managed by persons not trained in their understanding or resolution.

In any case, college psychiatrists tend to minimize the importance of making an early psychiatric diagnosis, emphasizing instead development of a sensitive understanding of all the issues leading up to the inhibiting emotional conflict. Students coming for help are not encouraged to think of themselves as sick persons, but instead as persons wise enough to seek better approaches to the resolution of their conflicts than they can achieve singlehanded. This part of a college psychiatrist's work may be considered as special tutoring in the area of emotional maturation and thus parallel and consistent with other tutors' efforts, which encourage the development of intellectual maturity. Of course, students with well-defined neuroses and psychoses are diagnosed as all other patients are, but the emphasis is placed on problem-solving within the educational framework rather than simply psychotherapy for an illness.

College students' emotional problems are often in the nature of life crises that respond quickly to professional help. Students usually react quite openly; their symptoms have not yet become fixed nor their defenses rigidified. Although establishing discrete categories helps to clarify discussion, in fact the categories overlap. Students must deal with the disruptions, dislocations and discontinuities inherent in any change of status, in addition to some that are peculiar to the college experience and their developmental stage. The stresses and the students' reactions to them are partly determined and largely affected by personality deficiencies (in which case the stresses may prove threatening, even overwhelming), and personality strengths (so that the same stresses mobilize students' abilities and improve their skills, thus helping them toward maturity).

Not only do many students not need longterm treatment—they don't want it. In fact, some may be reluctant to see a psychiatrist at all because they want to be completely independent. Students don't request psychiatric help lightly; when they *do* ask for help it is usually because they are very uncomfortable and feel they really need it. Students may see psychotherapy as a useful tool, perhaps one to be used *in extremis*, but they rarely consider it a source of prestige.

In general, college students are fairly sophisticated about psychiatry. They have some knowledge of psychiatric theory and practice, and tend to be psychologically-minded.

Students who are in emotional distress and who have no recourse to psychiatric help find other ways to express their disturbance: dropping out, academic failure, cheating, drinking, vandalism, drug use, inappropriate sexual behavior, etc. If they cannot talk out their problems they may act them out. The college psychiatrist's task is to aid such individuals in acquiring the needed insight to approach their problems more constructively.

To be effective, the college psychiatrist's value lies partly in what he is not—he is not a parent, dean, teacher, police officer, or student. He doesn't make administrative, legal or moralistic judgments. When a student comes to him voluntarily the student has already made the judgment that something is wrong, that in some way he is not doing his best or being the person he would like to be and believes he can be; he is demonstrating that he is aware of his emotional discomfort or his inefficiency. Thus the student makes the most important part of the diagnosis himself. Identifying the psychodynamics and helping the student to resolve his problems, to get where he wants to go in the most constructive manner, is the psychiatrist's job. Even with students who don't come voluntarily, the fact that the psychiatrist is not an agent for anyone except the student is important. This does not mean that the psychiatrist does not also represent the interests of the rest of the academic community and society at large; it does mean that his primary function is to be therapeutic.

The evaluation of the student who presents difficulties and the formulation of a tentative working diagnosis is in most instances therapeutic in itself. As already indicated, most college students are fairly sophisticated psychologically and are quick to recognize subtle forms of emotional conflict. To be sure, many of them are quite well informed about psychological theory, but have less awareness of how such knowledge may apply to them. If the psychiatrist underrates their intellectual grasp of an issue under examination and makes an authoritarian pronouncement that seems patronizing to the student, he can easily lose the confidence and respect of his patient. A sound rule for most college psychiatrists is to assume that their student patients are better informed and more capable intellectually than they themselves were at the patients' age.

For the most part, psychotherapy in college health services must be brief and the schedule arranged flexibly to take advantage of the student's readiness to learn about himself. In other words, a fixed schedule of one or two hours a week may result in inefficient use of time, but shorter periods arranged at or near the times of acute emotional stress may be more effective. If college psychiatrists attempt to give definitive treatment to all who need it, they will soon fill their schedules with such patients and have no time left for the essential tasks that only they can do.*

Although psychotherapy is the most important of the college psychiatrist's duties, the others that logically fall to him constitute the chief opportunity to develop constructive attitudes toward emotional problems. As critical situations arise in the day-to-day life of a college, the psychiatrist may be consulted by the administration because of student behavior that may suggest undue emotional stress, or concerning the suitability of some corrective measure instead of a punitive one. Admissions committees may seek his help on questions involving the capacity of a student to do satisfactory academic work; or an applicant with prior emotional problems may ask for an evaluation of his potential to perform satisfactorily in college. Student leaders may seek his assistance in organizing social service programs for the benefit of underprivileged groups in their communities.

Much of what a psychiatrist does in furthering emotional maturation among students can be equally well done by others, once those persons get the idea that it should be done. The psychiatrist's job is to ask questions about current practices that may not occur to others, particularly those relating to issues about which students have strong feelings and opinions. Furthermore, he should be readily available for consultation with all other members of the college who have responsibility for students and who are in quandaries about how they may help resolve issues with a strong emotional component.

It is essential that a college psychiatrist not become, or even appear to be, the agent of the administration against the students or of the students against the administration. His central concern is that of facilitating learning, and a major component of learning is responsibility. The maintenance of confidentiality is thus of essential importance. Although he must work with students, deans, presidents, counselors, police and security officials, he must be careful not to use his influence or knowledge unfairly. Some critics

---

*For a description of some of these tasks see pp. 17-20 of *Psychiatry, Education, and the Young Adult.*[10]

of college psychiatry doubt that a psychiatrist can work with all these persons without violating confidence (and usually that of students, they insist), but dozens of good health services are showing that it can be done.

The essential features of confidentiality in college health services (as well as industrial clinics) have recently been formulated by the Committee on Ethics of the American Psychiatric Association and approved by the appropriate councils of the American Psychiatric Association, American Medical Association and the American College Health Association.*

The general principles observed by most services include the following principles:

No confidential information is divulged without the patient's permission (with rare exceptions).

Psychiatric records are kept separate from other medical records and scrupulously protected. No one but physicians and specially authorized collaborators (social workers, psychiatrists, secretaries) have access to records.

Psychiatric records are never made available to admissions committees or security investigators.

Records should include only details necessary to understand the illness; omit minute details and names. "Write everything as though it will appear in court."

No information from records or other confidential sources is given to deans and other college administrators without written authorization by the patient. The administration is not informed of any infraction of rules.

Parents or next-of-kin are not informed that a student is receiving treatment unless hospitalization is necessary or the illness is of a very serious nature. In such instances, the patient is informed of what is to be done and why.

Psychiatric records are not used for screening purposes by other educational institutions nor by the graduate schools of the same university.

In rare instances, when a student's illness is so serious that his own life or the lives of others are endangered, it is sometimes necessary for the psychiatrist to take action against the patient's will or to supply information to the authorities. This serious step must never be taken except in genuine emergencies, and as a response to a real threat to life or safety.†

The psychiatrist also, of course, has a responsibility to the university at large. Thus, although he protects the confidentiality of the patient-physician

*Position Statement on Confidentiality and Privilege With Special Reference to Psychiatric Patients, *American Journal of Psychiatry,* 124:1015-1017, Jan. 1968.

†These and other principles are given in detail in *College Health Administration,*[7] pp. 72-78, and *Psychiatry, Education, and the Young Adult,*[10] pp. 188-199.

relationship, he does not protect the student from appropriate disciplinary measures. For this is not his job—it works against his job, because it is basically antitherapeutic, often seeming to excuse the student from the consequences of his actions. Psychiatric treatment or consultation is in no case a club that administration holds over the head of students, or that students can hold over the head of administration officials.

Those who plan college psychiatric services have to pay special attention to the needs of adolescents, even though entrance to college theoretically symbolizes the attainment of adulthood. To assume that all students are capable of acting in an adult manner is too high a compliment to pay in many instances. But to assume that undergraduates are still adolescents is unfair and inappropriate. A workable compromise is to treat all undergraduates as mature individuals with the unexpressed reservation that many of them will need considerable guidance and support, perhaps even limits, for a while.

The stage of late adolescence or young adulthood is characterized by ambivalence and tensions—the desire to be like adults but occasional need to be like children. Childhood represents limits and restraints, but also safety and security; independence is challenging, but also threatening. Both energies and conflicts increase. Some can handle their emotions by sublimation, but others must "act out," and there is an increase in fantasy life and narcissism. Relationships with parents are of critical importance. Much effort is directed toward breaking away from them, but love still exists, though with less dependency. It is in this context that current problems and tasks have to be dealt with.

Among the numerous maturational issues are: changing from dependent to independent relationships with older people, learning to tolerate ambiguity, defining one's own being and values, learning to deal with authority, and attaining successful sexual identification.

The student in college is largely on his own. He must organize his life, establish priorities, make or postpone career choices, utilize effective study techniques. He must move away from his previous dependence on adults to a new independence; he must, in short, learn to be himself. Often, at the same time that he is doing this, his sense of alienation and impersonality is heightened. This may come from a previous lack of feelings of acceptance; it is often due to the increasing size and complexity of universities. Among the vast computerization and milling throngs of people it becomes more and more difficult to find friends, to sort out values, to have personal contact with faculty and other trusted adults. In college, also, the student first meets the hard realities of political and social conditions which may undermine his belief in the importance and power of the individual, or cause him to give up faith in the solution of social and cultural problems.

Often he is confronted with so many choices—about careers, goals, life styles, as well as the almost numberless daily decisions—that freedom often threatens to turn into chaos. Each choice, in ruling out other possibilities, looms as a kind of irreversible major decision, and the whole situation seems to be out of control. In many cases it is wisest for the student to impose a kind of "moratorium" on some of these choices and to learn to live with uncertainty and ambiguity about certain aspects of life. At the same time he must maintain his sense of effectiveness, purpose, defining and working towards goals.

It is no wonder that under all of this the student will sometimes manifest symptoms of rather severe stress. But symptoms of this kind often respond well to short-term counseling or psychotherapy. They are frequently not a sign of psychopathology, but rather a common human response to a multitude of uncertain factors. Identifying the significant elements producing inhibiting emotional conflict, together with an affirmation of the students' ability to cope with them (when appropriate), can often be helpful in a very short time.

In achieving a sense of competence, of esteem, of security in the midst of all the insecurities of his life, the student draws on past family experiences which should, during college, be internalized, made a part of himself. He needs intellectual stimulation, peer group approval, and the feeling that past, present and future do form a continuum of experience. This sense of selfhood gives him a reality which will reduce the stresses of transition. If he has been given good role models, if the values of his family and his teachers are ones which he can accept as his own, he has an even more secure base on which to work.

Along with the new freedom which college life brings comes the necessity of redefining one's relation to authority. Students can and often do try to reject all authority, proclaiming an "ethic of anarchy" and setting themselves up as the final judge of all things, a situation which leads to chaos in their own lives, and also chaos in the larger social structure of which they are a part. Impulsivity is also a characteristic of the age group, making self-control a very vital goal to obtain. Previous experiences affect the student's ability to practice self-control, and many students will feel that immediate gratification of feeling is more important than any hypothetical gain to be achieved in the future. Part of the educational process is to teach the weighing of present action and future goals and to decide rationally on a course of action.

Student impulsivity is notorious; students tore apart the great universities of the Middle Ages, and they have not stopped yet. From "panty-raid" types of group action to the law-defying student riots of the past two years, it is obvious that impulse control is one lesson which our young people find especially hard to learn. And yet this impulsiveness can be channeled into many socially constructive forms. The students who said, "The denial of civil rights to the Negro people is wrong; let us do something about it," have often been impulsive, demanding an immediate response, acting without thinking through all the consequences. But it cannot be denied that they accomplished positive actions which their calmer and more controlled elders, for all their talk and all their careful planning, had been unable to manage.

One of the most ubiquitous problems confronting students is a society which uses sex inappropriately—to stimulate consumption, as an antidote to loneliness, as a kind of immediate gratification with no obligation or commitment involved. Paradoxically, the society traditionally does not permit sexual relations outside of marriage; so young people are subjected to a constant stimulus with no approved gratification. The stresses involved are probably most intense in mid-adolescence, but they spill over into college.

Recently there has been a very constructive emphasis on the recognition and rejection of hypocritical standards and of avoiding the exploitation of other human beings. Sexual morality is changing its focus; it now involves a great deal more freedom and a great deal more responsibility. Students who have never learned that "freedom" does *not* mean "what you can get away with" must be taught to act responsibly in this area also, to see that a mature relationship with another person involves much more than sex, and that sexual activity is no magical cure for all the stresses and ambivalences in their lives.

As a background to the various clinical problems that arise among college students, several conditions in student lives stand out with almost predictable frequency.

Culture shock. If the college environment differs significantly from his own background, a student experiences stress. To some this is stimulating and widens their horizons; for others it produces anxiety because past assumptions and patterns are threatened or new styles require tremendous adjustment. Disparities between rural and urban life, religious and ethical orientations, conservative and liberal politics, etc., may produce "culture shock."

Quite often, students who come from a country with relatively few modern ideas concerning mental health develop emotional problems with psychosomatic symptoms as the primary disability. When they learn that they have no "physical" disease but that their symptoms are based on their emotional conflicts, they may be unwilling or unable to accept such a concept, implying that it is only the inadequacy of Western medicine or incompetence of the physician which prevents the "true" cause being found and treated. In such cases, aiding the individual to cope with his burdensome difficulties is far more important (and effective) than trying to convince him of the correctness of the diagnosis.

Parental conflict. In the cases of at least two-thirds of all students who seek help for their emotional problems, their own parents have appeared to them to be in conflict with one another. This may take many forms, but is particularly harmful when one of the parents has used the patient in order to fight the other.

Marked contrast in values between home and college background. Rapid social change tends to produce or increase vulnerability to emotional stress in anyone, but students may be made particularly susceptible when they must assume unusual academic responsibilities while at the same time reacting to fundamentally different social requirements.

Inadequate or improper role models. Students, like younger children, tend to imitate what they observe rather than follow precepts passed on to them with appropriate examples.

Extreme permissiveness or rigidity, or inconsistencies in discipline. As children must learn what they can get away with and what they cannot, so adolescents need definite standards to adopt or to struggle against. Illogical or inconsistent discipline very often will make a young person feel that there is no logic, consistency or reason behind a particular value system, and that his approach to ethical matters must be an impulsive response leading to immediate gratification.

Inadequate or improper sexual education. Overemphasis on physical sexual prowess, accompanied by inadequate teaching about the psychological and spiritual aspects of sexuality, leave many young people gravely concerned as to what is expected of them.

Failure of parents to perceive their children as separate individuals. Even young children respond to being treated with respect for their individual needs and feelings. They can tell when they are being used as objects of ego gratification. A student who is in college because his parents need children who reflect credit on them usually has unsound motivation.

Lack of meaning and purpose in what they have been doing. Children find learning enjoyable for its own sake. As adolescence ensues, the connection between present and future may appear more tenuous than formerly; hence, long-term purposes and goals are needed. The college student demands "relevance" between his college experience and what he hopes to become.

Poor study habits. Even the most capable students cannot maintain a high level of accomplishment unless they are frequently required to work up to capacity. As one wise teacher said, "The student who is never asked to do more than he can do will never do as much as he can."

Response to stress takes many forms. Among the most common is the development of altered physiological function resulting from emotional conflict, such as asthma, gastrointestinal symptoms, muscular aches and pains, or headache. All these, usually considered together as psychosomatic symptoms, form a considerable proportion of college students' discomforts. Many of them are treated in the general medical clinics; others are referred or go directly to the psychiatric service.

Certain constellations of problems appear with sufficient frequency to warrant special consideration. Among the most common in late adolescents and young adults are fear of homosexuality, as well as homosexuality itself, depression, apathy, suicide and the misuse of drugs.

The ambivalences, stresses and adjustment problems of the college student are usually manifested in one or more clinical problems. These are the actual symptoms with which the psychiatrist deals. The five most common among late adolescents are depression, apathy, suicide, fears of homosexuality, and drug use.

Depression is probably the most common symptom which causes students to seek help. About one-half of all students seen by psychiatrists at Harvard show some depression. The risk of suicide is always kept in mind with these patients, but in my opinion the development of a relationship of trust and confidence between the patient and his psychiatrist (or other counselor) is the single best preventive measure against suicide.

A precursor of depression noted in many students is a condition of decreased affect in which they appear lethargic, dull, indolent and totally disinterested in their academic work. They describe feelings of emptiness, indifference, physical lethargy and inadequacy. This syndrome has been called *apathy* by Walters, who outlined the psychodynamics involved.[24]

Suicide is always of acute concern to college psychiatrists and deans particularly because of the dramatic nature of this form of behavior. The people who attempt it are usually, though not always, depressed. Those who attempt suicide but do not succeed quite often recover their health completely, thus justifying heroic efforts to save their lives. About six students attempt suicide for every one who succeeds, but this estimate should have further study.

Accidents and suicides are the two main causes of death among college students. Whether the suicide rate among students is increasing is not known. At Harvard University there were 35 suicides from 1946 to 1965 but the rate was 50 per cent lower during the last seven-year period (coincident with the establishment of a comprehensive psychiatric service) as compared with the first twelve years.[10 ;pp. 83-93]

Blaine and Carmen have made a study of 69 suicide attempts at Harvard University from 1962 through 1967. Among male undergraduates the rate was 5.7 per 10,000, and among female undergraduates 12.7 per 10,000. Of the 69, 53 involved undergraduates (35 male, 18 female) and 16 were graduate students. Among the latter 9 were men, 7 were women, though the rate was 11 per 10,000 for men and 55 per 10,000 for women.

From the standpoint of management it was encouraging that 29 of the 69 were treated in the college infirmary and were able to return to their studies without leaving college. Of the 25 who were hospitalized, 3 were able to complete their school work without taking a leave of absence. The most striking findings were the high number who had recently suffered a severe loss of some kind or who were concerned about studying effectively.[4]

Homosexuality need not be a special problem any more than any other variation from accepted norms is a problem. This condition is considered as a medical problem, a matter of incomplete psychosexual development, and is treated as such. All other personality characteristics are taken into account; the work of the psychiatrist is to find out what the stresses are that have produced the particular symptom of homosexuality. In many cases administration officials, faced with a homosexual episode which previously would have meant expulsion or legal action for those involved, have come to see that this emotional reaction is quite unfounded, and are giving students the opportunity of receiving psychiatric treatment and working to solve their problems.

Fear of becoming a homosexual concerns many students intensely. They often interpret a relatively minor episode—a homosexual advance by an acquaintance, a feeling of deep attraction to someone of their own sex—as "proof" that they are homosexuals. They may come to the psychiatrist in very real terror concerning their sexual identity. His assurance that these occurrences are common, that everyone's sexuality is partially polarized, and that homosexual urges are usually nothing more than manifestations of adolescence not yet outgrown, can create a great sense of relief in the troubled student and improve his functioning with very great rapidity.

The use of drugs as a solution to one's personal emotional conflicts is an old custom, but until recently it has been largely confined to those whose personal and social lives have been grossly unsatisfactory. Members of minority groups who are the victims of unfair discrimination or gross poverty, together with those individuals whose personal problems have become greater than they could cope with successfully, have been the most frequent users of drugs to attain some measure of relief from or "oblivion" of their plight. In recent years, particularly the last decade, the term "drugs" has acquired a quite different connotation in the minds of many people. It brings up images of "freeing the mind," "exploration of inner space," "developing insight," or "enhancing creativity," to those who approve of their use. The hallucinogenic, psychedelic, psychotomimetic, or mind-distorting drugs (the label depends on one's point of view) include psilocybin, LSD (lysergic acid diethylamide), marijuana, and many others. Recently, the amphetamines, especially the stronger ones and those used in very large amounts, have been included in this new popular meaning of "drugs."

The incidence of use among college students varies from year to year and place to place depending upon many factors. The use of marijuana appears to be increasing, that of LSD decreasing, in most colleges. A recent survey of Yale and Wesleyan students indicated that about 20 per cent of all students had used hallucinogenic drugs, mainly marijuana.[17] The results are consistent with numerous unpublished informal surveys conducted by students at various colleges, including my own institution. A definite statement labeling marijuana as a dangerous drug, but deploring the unnecessarily harsh and unrealistic penalties for its use has recently been issued by committees of the National Research Council and the American Medical Association.*

Fortunately, most of the drugs used by college students are not physically addictive. They are, however, habituating and the amphetamines especially can cause rather severe body damage. More dangerous is the fact that the hallucinogenic drugs may cause serious mental disturbances and possible irreversible damage to the mind. At the least, marijuana can cause an inability to concentrate, study, or focus clearly on life problems. Other hallucinogens have all too often led to psychotic episodes of varying degrees of severity.

The college psychiatrist thus must be prepared to treat the pathological mental state brought on by drug abuse. But often the patient does not manifest any symptoms of illness and may insist strenuously that his drug use is not a negative but a positive factor in his life. The psychiatrist then has the difficult task of persuading him that his drug use represents an in-

---

*AMA Council on Mental Health and Committee on Alcoholism and Drug Dependence; and Committee on Problems of Drug Dependence of National Research Council, National Academy of Science, "Marijuana and Society," *JAMA*, 203:1181-1182, June 24, 1968.

ability to achieve satisfaction in his life. The mature individual should not need to use drugs in a nonmedical situation; those who are helping him achieve maturity must lead him to a place where drugs are no longer necessary to him.

I have already stated that if the only role of a psychiatrist on a college health service staff is to care for severely disturbed students and staff members, he is unnecessary, because this function could be equally well performed by a private psychiatrist in the community. The basic goal of a college mental health program is to help maintain the effectiveness of the educational pursuits of students and faculty and to deal with both personal and institutional factors which limit and interfere with the learning experience.

College psychiatry has developed, without its practitioners realizing it, as a prototype of what is now more familiarly known as "community psychiatry." Its basic premises are that its services shall be available to all who need them, that help should be provided as soon as possible (when it is most effective), and that every attempt should be made to keep the individual functioning in his own community with as few dislocations and disruptions as possible.

Other basic goals include:

1. Changing the attitudes of students, faculty and employees toward emotional problems from aversion, fear or denial, to understanding, tolerance and cooperation in their management.

2. Improving relations between students and college staff in order to increase educational effectiveness.

3. Freeing the intellectual capacity of students to do creative and satisfying work.

4. Identifying and counteracting anti-intellectual forces that impede or prevent learning.

5. Creating a complex network of communication among all departments in the institution to facilitate early discovery of signs of disabling conflict. This must be done without creating the impression that there is a spy system, even one established for benevolent purposes.

6. Coordinating and integrating all counseling services in the institution, not with a view to domination or control, but to see that all available resources are available to anyone needing them.

If college mental health programs, of which psychiatric services in college health centers constitute an essential element, are to achieve their purposes, a blend of activities is necessary; brief psychotherapy, management of acute emergencies, collaboration between psychiatrists and numerous other persons who have responsibility for students, and continuous study of those conditions within the college or university which foster or impair effective learning. All these must be done without violating privacy or breaking confidences.

The field of college psychiatry is only beginning to open up. Its practice is one of the most rewarding (in personal satisfactions) and hopeful of all the methods by which psychiatry can be helpful in the understanding and solution of the problems of our society.

REFERENCES

1. Blaine, G. B., Jr.: *Patience and Fortitude.* Boston, Atlantic-Little, Brown, 1962.
2. Blaine, G. B., Jr.: *Youth and the Hazards of Affluence.* New York, Harper and Row, 1966.
3. Blaine, G. B., Jr., and McArthur, C. C. (Eds.): *Emotional Problems of the Student.* New York, Appleton-Century-Crofts, 1961.
4. Blaine, G. B., Jr., and Carmen, L. I.: Causal factors in suicidal attempts by male and female college students. *Amer. J. Psychiat.* 1969, in press.
5. Erikson, E. H.: *Identity and the Life Cycle.* Selected papers, Psychological Issues 1:1. New York, International Universities Press, 1959.
6. Erikson, E. H.: *Identity—Youth and Crisis.* New York, W. W. Norton, 1968.
7. Farnsworth, D. L. (Ed.): *College Health Administration.* New York, Appleton-Century-Crofts, 1964.
8. Farnsworth, D. L.: *College Health Services in the United States.* Washington, The American College Personnel Association (Div. of American Personnel and Guidance Association), 1965.
9. Farnsworth, D. L.: *Mental Health in College and University.* Cambridge, Harvard University Press, 1967.
10. Farnsworth, D. L.: *Psychiatry, Education, and the Young Adult.* Springfield, Ill., C. C Thomas, 1966.
11. Fry, C. C.: *Mental Health in College.* New York, Commonwealth Fund, 1942.
12. Group for the Advancement of Psychiatry: *The Role of Psychiatrists in Colleges and Universities.* Report #17, revised Jan. 1957. New York, G. A. P. Publication Office.
13. Group for the Advancement of Psychiatry: *Considerations on Personality Development in College Students.* Report #32, May 1955. New York, G.A.P. Publication Office.
14. Group for the Advancement of Psychiatry: *The College Experience: A Focus for Psychiatric Research.* Report #52, May 1962. New York, G.A.P. Publication Office.
15. Group for the Advancement of Psychiatry: *Sex and the College Student.* Report #60, Nov. 1965. New York, G.A.P. Publication Office.
16. Group for the Advancement of Psychiatry: *Normal Adolescence: Its Dynamics and Impact.* Report #68, Feb. 1968. New York, G.A.P. Publication Office.
17. Imperi, L. L., Klever, H. D., and David, J. S.: Use of hallucinogenic drugs on campus. *JAMA* 204:87-91, June 1968.
18. Keniston, K.: *The Uncommitted.* New York, Harcourt, Brace and World, 1965.

19. Keniston, K.: *Student Radicals*. New York: Harcourt, Brace and World, 1968.

20. Pervin, L. A., Reik, L. E., and Dalrymple, M.: *The College Dropout and Utilization of Talent*. Princeton, N.J., Princeton University Press, 1966.

21. Sanford, N.: *Self and Society—Social Change and Individual Development*. New York, Atherton Press, 1966.

22. Sutherland, R. L. et al. (Eds.): *Personality Factors on the College Campus*. Austin, Texas, Hogg Foundation for Mental Health, 1962.

23. Usdin, G. L.: *Adolescence, Care and Counseling*. Philadelphia, J. B. Lippincott, 1967.

24. Walters, P. W., Jr.: Student apathy. *In* Blaine, G. B., Jr., and McArthur, C. C. (Eds.): *Emotional Problems of the Student*. New York, Appleton-Century-Crofts, 1961, pp. 153-171.

25. Wedge, B. M. (Ed.): *Psychosocial Problems of College Men*. New Haven, Yale University Press, 1958.

26. Whittington, H. G.: *Psychiatry on the College Campus*. New York, International University Press, 1963.

27. Yamamoto, K.: *The College Student and His Culture: An Analysis*. Boston, Houghton Mifflin, 1968.

Psychiatric Reactions to Accidents

HERBERT C. MODLIN, M.D.

THE BIBLE SAYS: "Be sure your sins will find you out." This ancient statement embodies a truth Medicine must ruefully acknowledge with reference to the term "traumatic neurosis"; for the unwitting past sin of alluding to certain syndromes under that loose designation persistently haunts us despite our efforts now to disavow its validity. We begat "traumatic neurosis," and unfortunately the law adopted our illegitimate waif, gave him a home, and has come to love him as its own.

The Standard Nomenclature of Diseases, published by the American Medical Association, does not list "traumatic neurosis." It is not an officially recognized diagnostic label although it has been part of our medical jargon since World War I. As jargon, it is used by physicians and attorneys to express too wide a variety of meanings for inclusion in one generally accepted definition.

The basic idea connoted by "traumatic neurosis" is not altogether invalid. Sudden accidents can precipitate psychiatric illnesses. Why then not use the term? For several reasons it can be inexact and misleading.

In standard medical vocabulary, "trauma" refers to tissue damage. We have adapted the word to psychiatric terminology and commonly speak of "psychic trauma" to convey the idea that the human mind as well as the human body can be hurtfully affected by external assaults. Confusion will reign unless the exact context of "trauma" is articulately defined. This applies particularly in medico-legal communication since many jurisdictions still do not accept the concept of psychic trauma and do not allow recovery for injury unless there has been some damage to or at least a contact with the physical body of the victim. Such rulings in effect deny the reality of the mind, of psychopathology and of psychiatry.

Since neurosis is a psychic rather than a somatic disturbance, it follows that the stress or trauma which triggers it must be psychic. Physical injury

Sections of this paper have been taken from the following publications:

Modlin, H. C.: The post-accident anxiety syndrome: Psychosocial aspects. *Amer. J. Psychiat.* 123:1008-12, 1967.

Modlin, H. C.: Psychiatric reactions to accidents. *Washburn Law J.* 6:317-323, 1967.

itself does not, cannot alone produce a neurosis. A fractured bone does not cause a phobia; a sprained back cannot cause a depression. Both physical and psychological injury may result from the same accident, and physical injury may foster subsequent unconscious neurotic conflict. Patients may suffer a severe psychological reaction to loss of a limb, a disfigured face or a period of intractable pain, but in each case it is the psychological meaning of the physical damage which lights up a neurotic process.

The second word of our suspect phrase can also lead to confusion. In psychiatric nosology, "neurosis" has specific meaning. There are six definable kinds of neuroses; and many of the disabling psychological consequences of accidents are not actually neuroses at all. Then, too, in a psychodynamic sense, all neuroses are traumatically induced or engendered, an idea that compounds our semantic dilemma.

The common sense and legal implications in "traumatic neurosis" unduly emphasize a single traumatic event as the proximate cause of illness, thus nullifying one of the axioms of psychological science—multiple causality. Some two million persons were injured last year in auto accidents, almost that many in industrial accidents, and many more than that number in home accidents; yet only a small percentage of these millions developed incapacitating psychiatric reactions. Why did those few? We postulate a predisposition, a personality defect or weakness which made these people unduly susceptible to that particular kind of life event. Also, other circumstances in the current life of each victim at the time of the psychological trauma frequently contribute to the chain of causal events; for example, an uncomfortable work situation or a failing marriage. The legal concept of sole proximate cause is uncongenial to medical science.

Enough of worrying this phrase in the manner of a dog with a meatless bone. If I am unhappy with "traumatic neurosis," what then do I suggest as communicative phraseology? Let me speak from here on about psychiatric reactions to accidents, and discuss with you four points: (1) the kinds of syndromes we commonly see following accidents; (2) the role of the accident as a precipitating event; (3) the course of illness; and (4) the reliability of medical knowledge and opinion concerning these reactions as a basis for legal decisions, such as disability and compensation.

SYNDROMES

The symptom constellations commonly resultant to accidents are anxiety reaction, conversion reaction, psychophysiologic reaction and dependency reaction. There should be no significant problem of assigning diagnostic labels. Our standard nomenclature is quite adequate for classification purposes and we see no unique specific syndromes for which we need a coined phrase such as traumatic neurosis. One variety of anxiety reaction (one possible exception) is a discrete, easily recognized set of symptoms which, in our experience, occurs only after sudden, unexpected accidents.

The component parts of the syndrome are all subjective complaints voiced by the patient and/or his family. Objective findings are minimal and the diagnosis rests on accurate history taking. It is exceedingly important to interview the spouse and other close family members since, characteristically, the patient is concrete, unimaginative, verbally unproductive and a poor observer of his own feelings and behavior.

1. *Anxiety.* The patients regularly describe chronic free-floating anxiety; "Something is about to happen." Many suffer acute uneasiness when unable to avoid circumstances which recall the accident such as hearing the hiss of steam, climbing a ladder, entering congested traffic, returning to the site of the accident.

2. *Muscular tension.* Symptomatic complaints are restlessness, fatigability, insomnia, impatience and the pervasive, "I just can't seem to relax."

3. *Irritability.* Hypersensitivity to noise and commotion is most vividly demonstrated in (a) the well-known startle reaction to sudden noises and (b) inability to tolerate the noise of the offspring at home. Frequently, the radio, television or conversation of well-meaning friends will occasion an irritable lashing out or withdrawal.

4. *Impaired concentration and memory.* Psychological tests demonstrate no real memory loss; subjective complaints of this altered mental functioning result from self-preoccupation and inattention to extra-ego matters.

5. *Repetitive nightmares,* directly or symbolically reproducing the experienced accident.

6. *Sexual inhibition.* A notably lowered interest in sexual relations regularly develops and may proceed to complete impotence or frigidity.

7. *Social withdrawal.* Avoidance of interpersonal involvement with relatives, friends, neighbors, clubs, church, recreation, the job, traffic—"Peace and quiet at any price."

Here is a clinical vignette: The car a 52 year old man was driving in a midwestern town at dusk stalled on some railroad tracks. In attempting to start the car, he flooded the engine. As he sat there waiting for the excess gasoline to drain out of the carburetor, a slowly moving switch engine suddenly appeared. The motorist had eight or ten seconds to grip the steering wheel and watch the one-eyed monster bear down on him. He received no physical injury from the impact which nudged the car off the tracks, but he was so affected by the experience that his legs buckled when he got out of the car. When he came to us eight months later, the patient complained of fearfulness, tension, restlessness, tearfulness, insomnia, nightmares, impaired concentration, irritability, loss of sexual capacity. He had lost twenty pounds in weight and had been dismissed from his job. Most of us would have been considerably shaken psychologically by such an experience, but most of us would have recovered in a few days or a week. For this man, the accident was disaster.

The conversion reaction usually consists of symptoms referable to the body site of physical injury. Simple suggestibility is a prominent mechanism.

Clinical example: A careless workman kicked a ten pound sandbag off the third floor of a construction job. It struck a man at work on the ground level, knocking him down. An hour later, the victim's shoulder pain made continued work impossible, and he was examined by the company physician. No serious injury could be discovered. After a week of physiotherapy, he was deemed ready for work. He returned to the job with a torticollis, his chin fixed over his left clavicle; but further examination revealed no physical explanation for the distorted position. The disability was finally relieved by one hypnotic session.

Clinical example: A 55 year old carpenter, stepping back to admire a completed piece of work, fell into an excavation hole behind him. Devoid of breath momentarily, he lay limply while other workmen gathered around the edge of the twelve feet deep hole and cautioned him not to move "because something might be broken." He was raised by an improvised stretcher and transported to the nearest physician. Cursory examination revealed considerable back pain and absent patellar reflexes; and the patient was sent by ambulance to the medical center nearby. Unfortunately, he shared a double room with a multiple sclerosis patient; and when examined an hour after admission he was paralyzed from the waist down.

The major disability in such patients usually arises from therapeutic neglect. If the symptoms remain unalleviated and secondary gain of illness sets in; if the limp or blindness or aphonia or torticollis become part of a picture of chronic invalidism; then remedial help is hard to apply. As a rule of thumb, if such symptomatology obtains for as long as two years, prognosis is poor.

The psychophysiological reaction, that peculiar interweaving of psyche and soma, is the postaccident condition least amenable to successful management. The persistent low back pain, the chronic syndrome, the "cardiac neurosis"—these are the most refractory problems.

The laborer lifts a heavy load: "something snaps"; pain develops quickly. Soft tissue injury is diagnosed and proper orthopedic treatment instituted. After six months the orthopedist states that the tissues should be well healed and he can no longer explain the patient's persistent pain and work disability on the basis of organic mechanisms. Eventually, the patient may appear for psychiatric evaluation; and, in turn, we may have difficulty in presenting a convincing explanation for his disability on purely psychiatric grounds. The probable factor of secondary gain may loom large, but the primary mechanisms remain obscure.

Dependency reaction, i.e., the exacerbation of a latent passive-dependent solution to stress, may appear in relatively pure culture or may complicate any of our other clinical observations. One common characteristic of these people we may label "inadequate." They are psychologically underdeveloped.

Clinical example: A forty year old plasterer fell eight feet to a terrazzo floor when his scaffold collapsed unexpectedly. Badly frightened by the experience, he stopped work. When on the following day he consulted a physician because of leg pain, the findings were essentially negative except for a linear fracture of the right os calcis requiring no specific treatment.

The patient sought psychiatric evaluation two years later because of his persistent inability to work and the chronic diffuse pain in both legs and hips unconfirmed by any physical findings. He lived with his widowed mother who devoted much attention to his welfare.

While on training maneuvers during World War II, he twisted a knee and spent the next year in army hospitals. He was unable to work for an additional year after discharge from military service. In 1955, gastric symptoms were diagnosed as a pre-ulcer state and diet and medication prescribed. An acute perforation of the stomach, which subsequently occurred, required only simple closure; but he could not work for eighteen months thereafter.

This seemingly uncomplicated man struggled through life at a marginal level of adjustment. At a casual, uncritical glance one might view him as an undistinguished but stable member of society. Closer inquiry reveals a sixth grade education; pathetically awkward and fruitless approaches to women; continued dependence on his mother and, when necessary, on his steadily employed brother. Such a person tends to stimulate irritation or contempt of physicians, insurance companies and the general public. He may be called lazy, dishonest, mercenary, etc. These are not sufficient explanations of his behavior for psychiatrists, nor should they be. Human psychology is not that simple.

THE ACCIDENT

Any kind of accident, life-threatening or inconsequential, may trigger one of the psychopathologic reactions mentioned above. The unexpected, potentially dangerous, near miss, in the absence of physical damage to the victim, usually triggers the anxiety reaction. The scaffold collapses, the steam pipe bursts, the crane tips over, the gasoline fumes flare into a flash fire. A construction worker I examined recently was blown off a roof by a passing helicopter. Any of these untoward experiences would undoubtedly produce at least a degree of psychic disequilibrium in even normal persons like you and me.

Minor accidents—the bump on the head, the pratfall—usually produce a psychophysiologic reaction: the aching back, the recurrent headache, the palpitation and dyspnea, the weak legs, the dizzy spells. A 35 year old woman slipped and fell in a sitting position on a ramp in a department store. When we examined her one year later she was tense, hypersensitive, tearful and unable to work because of diffuse low back pain unexplained by findings of repeated orthopedic examinations. This type of valid postaccident disability is difficult for the average man to understand and credit; he is prone to suspect malingering.

As a generality, there is a compensatory relationship between physical and psychic damage. The more extensive the tissue damage—fractures, lacerations, contusions, hemorrhage—the less likely a postaccident psychiatric disorder. Significant physical damage seems to bind or neutralize the reactive anxiety or depression that the patient might reasonably be expected to exhibit; he has something "real" to cope with instead of something intangible. The medical and nursing ministrations; the bed rest; the traction harness and plaster cast; the sedatives, analgesics and narcotics; the acceptable, even required, temporary state of regressed invalidism; the visible evidence of "battle" injury to display; the legitimate, socially condoned period of convalescent disability—all these factors tend to deter and inhibit the development of a neurotic complex of symptoms.

Conversely, a sudden, frightening accident with little or no physical damage is more often a precipitant of psychiatric disorders. After the fact, the traumatized psyche is not put at rest between cool white sheets; the hyperirritable nervous system is not soothingly bandaged and poulticed and fed intravenously; the invisible ego laceration is not legal tender for special consideration; and the victim's desire to retreat temporarily from the everyday stress of life is not socially approved. Incidentally, all these psychological treatments: immediate rest, sedation, isolation, enforced quiet, special attention under empathic medical authority, are being routinely encountered by our disturbed soldiers in Viet Nam with a resultant remarkably low incidence of psychiatric casualties. It is unfortunate that we have been unable to apply these hard-taught lessons of military psychiatry more tellingly to counterpart civilian problems.

COURSE OF ILLNESS

Once precipitated by an accident, the course of the syndrome can be influenced by a variety of factors, two of which are the quality and quantity of the precipitating accident and the strengths and weaknesses of a given patient's psychological equipment.

The havoc consequent to a severe precipitating stress depends upon the intrinsic strength of the target personality. The weaker the adaptive capacity of the psyche, the less the insult necessary to unbalance it. The more sudden and potentially dangerous the accident, the more likely it is to be psychologically unsettling—especially to an already teetering balance. A young man was involved in a headon collision and miraculously escaped physical injury. The girl riding with him was killed and a passenger in the other car was seriously injured. His postaccident anxiety and depression are easy to understand since that particular precipitating stress would be difficult for the most stable among us to tolerate with unruffled poise.

It follows that observers, using a common-sense frame of reference, are puzzled by, if not suspicious of the considerable disability some persons manifest after seemingly minor or even trivial accidents. Their skepticism is based on conviction that life consists only of what can be seen, that all people are approximately alike ("like me" is the usual point of comparison) and that *a* cause produces *an* event. For psychological science, all these propositions are in error. People vary greatly in their personality strengths and weaknesses; and the capacity for flexible tolerance the victim brings with him to the accident must be duly considered as one determinant of his postaccident recovery from its psychological impact. "One man's meat is another man's poison." What appears to an observer a minor stress may constitute a major psychic assault to a given victim's uniquely vulnerable arrangement of internal resources and the particular set of external circumstances that happen at the time to be impinging upon him. We may well be unaware that the so-called accident victim was already near his breaking point because of antecedent stresses unknown to us and even, possibly, not consciously recognized by the victim himself. The accident, then, can be a "last straw" phenomenon.

Many patients who become ill, inadvertently and unconsciously discover a certain secondary gain in being a patient. The suffering from symptoms and the position of invalidism may seem a solution (albeit second rate) to certain life problems. The 55 year old construction worker may be able to push out of consciousness his slowly fading physical strength, his diminishing muscular agility, his increasing weariness at the end of the day, his mildly waning sexual powers. He needs to believe "I am as good a man as I ever was," and "experience is what counts on my job." He needs to maintain self-respect and self-esteem, to deny how he is struggling to keep pace with the vigorous 23 year old apprentice working beside him on the same job. When this man suffers a sprained back, a bruised shoulder, a period of heat exhaustion in midsummer, a brief episode of coma from a minor blow to the head, his unconscious coping processes are presented with a legitimate, face-saving way out of a troubling situation. Thus a protective, problem-solving invalidism may set in. This is an example of a psychological maneuver commonly seen. In medicine it may complicate any illness—medical, surgical, obstetrical, psychiatric—and is not peculiar to postaccident reactions. In fact, this psychological mechanism of solving Problem A by succumbing to Problem B is a universal phenomenon of human behavior not peculiar alone to beneficiaries of medical and/or legal expertise.

The 35 year old woman previously mentioned was married to a crippled watch repairman fifteen years her senior. At eighteen, she had left an uncomfortable family situation to earn a living as a waitress. She was clerking in an Army P.X. when she met her future husband. He hired her as an assistant, taught her his trade, and eventually they married. At the time of her accident, she was spending six to eight hours a day on a watchmaker's stool; then more hours managing their house. The couple had no children and no social life. The painful coccyx resulting from her fall effectively separated the pair part of the day and also necessitated a moratorium of their sexual relations to which she had never adjusted.

An oil well troubleshooter, married and with three children, earned a comfortable living for his family through his expertness at returning faltering wells to production, frequently collected overtime pay since he and his small crew were on call day and night. The work was often hazardous, but the patient accepted all job assignments and pursued them with conscientious thoroughness. At one difficult job on a freezing, snowy night in January, the patient slipped and fell twice from a truck, landing in a sitting position each time. He gave up and pulled his crew off the job for the first time in years. Incapacitating low back pain set in, became chronic and he was "forced" to leave the oil wells for much less remunerative work as a salesman.

Intertwined factors further influencing prognosis in postaccident cases are the medical and the legal management of the patient/client. For the sake of brevity, I shall not review with you the things we do that we consider successful on the assumption that those cases not satisfactorily responsive to ordinary handling are the riddle all of us in common are more interested in seeking to solve.

In our experience, it is unusual for the psychiatrist to see a patient with a postaccident psychiatric syndrome until he has been examined by at least five physicians, sometimes eight or nine. Since in these illnesses as in most illnesses, early treatment offers the best chance for recovery, it is regrettable indeed that a great many patients are referred to us, for the first time, from six months to three years after the accident. It is also noteworthy that the large majority of referrals are by attorneys; although they may have received hints of psychic disorder from medical reports. These observations illustrate some of the problems of medical management. Obviously, the patients we do see are a special type, those whose psychiatric symptoms persist over a period of time and are not relieved by routine medical treatment.

One unfortunate aspect of what, in a sense, might be called medical mismanagement is a byproduct of legal operations. Most of the physicians who see these patients are, in legal terminology, examining rather than treating doctors, some brought into the case by the plaintiff's attorney, others by the defendant's. We are familiar with the concept of overtreatment; in too many of these patients overexamination has occurred. An unintentional sequel to such repeated examinations, usually with few or no findings of physical illness, may be that each medical report, "There's nothing much wrong with you," and meant to be reassuring, simply drives the patient further into his psychiatric illness. He displays his symptoms repetitively as a signal of psychic distress and an indirect cry for help.

Early recognition of the psychiatric factor in postaccident disability is crucial since, as a rule of thumb, when the conversion (hysterical) symptoms and the psychophysiologic (psychosomatic) symptoms continue unabated for two years, chances for recovery become seriously limited. In some of these cases, medicine and law, like two uncertain outfielders, have allowed the ball to drop between them, because neither player has seen a clear indication that he should assume responsibility for the play. As the patient passes from specialist to specialist, the plaintiff's attorney may find himself inadvertently in the role of medical coordinator, a most uncomfortable position. This general situation can be worsened by the traditional skepticism and delaying tactics of the defense. In such confusion the patient is always the loser.

A final question to consider is whether or not we in medicine, and psychiatry in particular, can assist the law in the determination of disability and the awarding of appropriate compensation in such multiply-victimized cases. From the standpoint of psychiatric knowledge, we answer "yes," and I have tried to explain in the foregoing the ordinary clinical bases of our potential helpfulness. From the standpoint of medical practice, we should answer "not always."

The effectiveness of the physician in contributing to the disposition of personal injury legal issues depends first on his willingness and interest in becoming involved in the tasks of the law. As you know, many physicians, perhaps the majority, are not willing. Secondly, the effectiveness of the physician depends on the ability of the lawyer to understand the frame of reference within which his medical colleagues must perform and the astuteness of the attorney in instructing his medical expert witness about a physician's functions within the legal arena.

As a psychiatrist, I see working in and with the law as an exercise in community psychiatry. In consultation with an attorney, in testifying before a Workmen's Compensation Commissioner, in a written report to an attorney or court, or in an appearance on the witness stand, I try to maintain the position of consultant. I accept the task of working with a nonmedical social institution concerned with plaintiffs or clients rather than patients, an institution that does not operate in the framework of health and illness. I am there to assist the court, the attorneys, the jury, the commissioner in their doing their job ably, by elucidating the mental health aspects of a legal problem. Correspondingly, I would hope that the attorney, the insurance carrier, the Compensation Commissioner would, at appropriate times, see it as their obligation to help me with my appointed social task of treating patients' illnesses.

The quite separate social functions that Law and Medicine serve rarely need be considered antithetical or competitive. If we can but be men of good will, our social functions can be complementary in cooperative help to the distressed people we both serve.

A New Look at Psychotherapeutic Evolution

LAWRENCE C. KOLB, M.D.

It is to Perry Talkington that I am indebted for the suggestion to take a new look at psychotherapeutic evolution, since it was almost fifteen years ago that I brought together the material for the Hutchings lecture, "Psychotherapeutic Evolution and its Implications." It was my wish, in developing that lecture,[8] to demonstrate the means by which a specific theoretical model of psychotherapy—psychoanalysis—had been used as a structure upon which various technical variations in the psychotherapeutic process had evolved in the treatment of a variety of psychopathologic entities. At that time, it was possible to draw from the work of the lonely innovators useful technical variations applicable to the treatment of schizophrenic reactions, manic depressive reactions and certain antisocial behavioral disturbances. These technical variations had come about through these innovators' perception of the fact that the analytic technique, primarily evolved from and adapted to treat certain neuroses, was inadequate in its basic processes in treatment of the psychoses. Accordingly, they courageously abandoned the insistent tenets of tradition-bound psychoanalysts, reexamined the psychopathology and empirically applied new technical variations. In the course of their efforts, we have learned much of the pathologic processes of development of personality in schizophrenia and the manic depressive reactions. From personal experience, reading the literature and observation of some of my friends' successful behavior in treating certain patients with these disturbances, it seemed possible to extract certain relatively clear distinctions in the therapeutic processes that may be specifically stated for use to all who wish to attempt their application in these conditions. These statements (articulated distinctions in psychotherapeutic technique) have been applied personally as general guidelines in treatment of patients with these serious conditions; they have also been useful in teaching residents and psychoanalytic students supervised by me.

Since the writing of the original lecture, there has occurred both the important introduction of the new pharmaceuticals for treatment and a vast expansion of our knowledge of those neurophysiologic processes pertaining to emotion and its modulation, as well as enlargement of our theoretical constructs—particularly as they relate to the psychogenesis of schizophrenia—and new ventures in treatment—particularly in family therapy.

As one looks at the scene today—over a quarter of a century after the extensive efforts at evolution of a rational psychotherapy for schizophrenia—one must first question the relationship of psychotherapy in the psychotic states to the administration of the psychopharmaceuticals. The issues here are several. The first and most commonly declared offers the pragmatic challenge. Is there any practical value in the use of intensive psychotherapy for psychoses when there is now available a number of highly potent pharmacologic agents capable of modifying pathologic behavior. Another issue often posed by those most dedicated to pursuit of psychotherapeutic process doubts the propriety of simultaneous use of that process with administration of pharmaceuticals. The assertion is made that the psychotherapeutic process is impeded when the therapist prescribes medications which alleviate the anxieties of the patient. Yet, still another position asserts that alleviation of the pathologic affect characteristic of the psychoses by administration of drugs makes it possible for many more patients to engage in a psychotherapeutic process. True, combined treatment is believed to lead in turn to new learning, better insight and, therefore, more certain behavioral change and social adaptability. None of these positions is supported by data with any certainty.

The attempt made in this discussion to distinguish different psychopathologies, their genesis and the appropriate psychotherapeutic variations derives from an outlook which emphasizes the philosophic importance of discovering the testing differences to bring about evolution. This attempt contrasts with Masserman's or Kiev's comparative studies of the similarities of the psychotherapeutic process used by different healers as viewed over historical time or between existing cultures.[7,9]

Jerome Frank has distilled these universal elements of psychotherapy in his definition of that process: "A series of more or less structured series of contacts between the healer and sufferer through which the healer, often with the aid of the group, tries to produce certain changes in the sufferer's emotional state, attitudes, and behavior. All concerned believe these changes will help him. Although physical and chemical adjuncts may be used, the healing influence is primarily exercised by works, acts, and rituals in which sufferer, healer and—if there is one—group participate jointly."[2]

Valuable as these efforts have been in definitions of the essential elements found in all forms of psychotherapy, the search for the rudimentary processes indigenous in every effort of the past is unlikely to achieve those discriminations of effort capable of evolution through new knowledge and theory building. It is the latter which have gained for us in so many of our endeavors those great advances in the health sciences.

Modern psychotherapy, in almost all its forms (aside from behavior therapy), has received its impetus from the construction of a well defined theory of personality coupled with a precisely articulated series of statements in regard to a technique of treatment—that is, psychoanalysis. If its practice has not spread widely beyond large urban areas, it has been well described, discussed and even attempted beyond the circles of established psychoanalytic practice. Using the psychoanalytic model, whether one considers it crude, poorly constructed, often ineffective or even offensive, it is possible to build and test many variations, describe their differences from the original and examine the applicability of the modified variants in numerous situations.

Psychoanalytic therapy has a more ambitious aim than alleviation of symptoms: to bring about a change in the personality structure of the patient so that, at the termination of treatment, he is not only symptom-free, but is capable of facing the internal and the environmental stresses that were conducive to the production and maintenance of the previous illness without again succumbing to the illness. If one accepts the additional tenet inherent in psychoanalytic concepts, that the series of interpersonal events occurring between parent and child are determinative to a large extent in the development of abnormal behavior disturbance, the reconstructed analytic patients should also have the potential of rearing children free of such illness. The analytic aims include not only therapy for the patient but concepts for the prevention of illness, both for the patient in the future and for the patient's offspring.

Attainment of these ambitious aims through psychoanalytic therapy depends (as its originator, Freud, pointed out so clearly in his paper, "Analysis Terminable and Interminable") on a balance of factors including the constitutional makeup of the individual, the importance of trauma in inducing the neurotic state, and the success of the analytic process in replacing insecure repressions and defenses by certain and egosyntonic controls. As he stated, "we may say that analysis is always right in theory in its claim to cure neurosis by insuring control over instinct but that in practice its claim is not always justified." This is not surprising for the power of analysis is not infinite: it is limited "and the final results always depend on the relative strength of the conflicting cyclical agencies."[3]

The theoretic aims of psychoanalytic therapy are important to keep in mind. First of all, these ambitious goals are those that all of us might agree we wish and desire for all our patients as the result of any treatment methods in psychiatry. Secondly, the stating of the goal makes it possible to evaluate the potential effectiveness of a treatment against the goal as well as the potential of other treatments against that goal. Too often in the evaluative efforts which have one form of treatment to another, evaluators fail to recognize, even to demand or search for, the goals the therapists propose to achieve. Comparisons which do not identify differences in goals are hardly useful in providing assessment for either the members of the profession or the public. Nor can they be considered as conducted by a scientific mind.

Perception of a goal establishes for therapists important and subtle differences in his attitude toward, and potentials for, appropriate psychotherapeutic management of patients with widely differing pathology. This is as it should be. The treating physician's attitude, intensity of contact, decision to use pharmaceutical aids and other means of treatment (expectations toward patients with such varying conditions as acute lobar pneumonia and chronic rheumatoid arthritis) are significant in the eventual outcome of treatment. Unrealistic goal expectations of the psychiatrist who undertakes treatment of a schizophrenic reaction, derived from his former expectations in managing neurotic phobic states, often spell disaster—for himself and his patient.

A critical essay of the therapeutic effectiveness of the various somatic therapies, including that provided by the pharmacological agents, shows only that they provide alleviation of symptoms. This alleviation may be interpreted as secondary to a quantitative reduction in affect, not as an expression of qualitative modification of the personality structure. Quantitative changes, however, are the more easily attained, and even if not permanent, may be distributed to a wider range of disturbed persons.

As a means of providing a framework for the discussion of specific technical modifications (and at the risk of exposing the reader to ennui), a brief review description of the essential elements of psychoanalytic technique will be given—as it was developed originally for treatment of the neuroses.

Briefly, the salient feature of the psychoanalytic technique is the systematic investigation of the transference relationship and the resistances of the patient, observed in treatment. As you know, this means the systematic examination of the patient's perception of the physician and the patient's ongoing emotional responses to him. By describing this relationship and then associating to it in terms of experiences with others, the patient is frequently surprised to find how he has distorted the physician in terms of the way he has learned to see others. From the repeated confrontation of such distortions of reality in a single individual in a usually neutral environment, the patient then may learn to discriminate more clearly the multifaceted personal contacts of his daily environment. Then he responds with emotions appropriate to the real transaction rather than with the ingrained and overdetermined repetitiveness laid down as the result of unfortunate past experiences. Resistance may be considered an expression of the ongoing interpersonal relationship with the therapist, a false perception of the therapist as someone who will respond unfavorably if the patient utters or acts out the unspeakable—isolated and buried in the unconscious. For this therapeutic process to succeed, the patient needs to maintain an ongoing feeling of security in his relationship with the therapist, a relationship necessary for any successful psychotherapy. This security, as in all other psychotherapies, sustains him on emergence of anxiety and hostility when these appear.

The processes of free association and dream analysis are techniques used to lead the patient to the experiences which determine his falsifications of current reality—the intimidating experiences which he has repressed and forgotten. All the other aspects of psychoanalytic practice such as the supine position, the formal relationship with the therapist, are subsidiary to the basic processes mentioned. They make it possible to maintain the analyst as a neutral figure and assist in bringing to the fore the distorting perceptual processes of the patient and this limited and repetitive infantile and child-like behavior in society.

Some insist that interpretation is an essential part of the psychoanalytic technique; there are others who have questioned its salient position in the psychoanalytic process. Certain personal observations bring me to question the preeminent position of verbal interpretation by the psychoanalyst in resolution of the transference distortions, the nuclear process of successful treatment. Some distortions are certainly worked through on nonverbal levels of communication. In the course of the treatment of the neurotic, the origin of each behavior trait, each repetitive thought process or somatic disturbance, is sought in this framework.

The ultimate aim of treatment carries with it eventual emancipation from the physician. Sometimes this final aim is unfulfilled. The patient may appear to function well in society; yet the physician is aware that a persistent dependency exists, or in some instances, that a distant but chronic paranoid relationship continues—although therapy is terminated. These are the end stages of many apparently successful and unsuccessful analytic ventures in treatment of the psychoneuroses.

Let us now turn to the psychotherapy of the schizophrenics. That therapy now has a firmer dynamic for its technique as we have come to appraise more critically the many forces which shape ego functioning. As Ives Hendricks[5] so clearly understood and described some 30 years ago, the schizophrenic suffers from a major impairment in ego functioning. There are the well known abnormalities in perception, thought and action, the latter being expressed particularly in efforts at communication, the capacity to evaluate reality and make judgments, to solve problems and adapt to reality. (Affect is seriously disturbed.) But today we recognize more sharply the lack of development of ego attitudes, of trust, autonomy, initiative and persistence. Their deficient growth is overshadowed by the contrasting attitudes of suspiciousness, mistrust, pathologic apathy and withdrawal and personal doubting, including uncertainties in both sexual and adult roles. Superego growth is also abnormal in the sense that oppressive inhibitions and restrictions exist in regards to expressions of aggressive sexual and dependency wishes. Likewise, the aspirational demands (expressions of the ego ideal) often exceed the individual talent, opportunity, and the time demands available for needed learning and experience.

The genesis of these ego and superego abnormalities cannot now be ascribed simply to the acquisition of the pathological defenses through the family transactional processes. To be sure, such transactions exist. We have good reason to believe that many of the impairments of ego functioning are the result of defective learning of the process of socialization, including communication, and the progressive differentiation of percepts so that one may properly assess reality. These deficiencies take place through the deprivation and isolation of the schizophrenic person within a particular family milieu or as a result of lack of appropriate stimulation early in life from parents or parental substitutes. We recognize, then, an early and ongoing depriving series of interactions: object relations are tenuous, inconstant and confusing.

Affect is held rigidly under control except when the highly constructed but limited repertoire of psychological defenses fail in the face of intense arousal. The defenses remain unbalanced by the development of realistically perceived and gratifying ego adaptive functions. Here I refer to the development of social and sexual vocational and avocational talents that are assessed correctly and which, in their exercise, afford personal pleasure. The lack of these ego functions is perhaps more often the result of experient lack of contact with family or other person relations with whom the patient can identify and from whom he can learn.

It may well be that the biological apparatus concerned with affective expression and its control are abnormally determined through genetic or constitutional grounds. There is some evidence to support this view. But, if true, it in no way obviates the necessity to have an understanding of the ongoing view of life experiences of the growing schizophrenic as these establish the characteristically human aspects of his total adaptation—the areas in which he fails. Correction here may do much to make him a functioning man or woman.

The establishment of a working relationship with the patient is the cornerstone of the therapy of the schizophrenic. The relationship of the patient to the therapist is of a different quality than that seen in neuroses. It is exceedingly fragile and is subject to withdrawal on the basis of any suspicion or indication that there is a limitation of interest on the part of the physician. Breaking through to obtain the trust of the severely suspicious, ill, nontrusting, withdrawn, highly sensitive and disturbed patient—who has not committed himself to treatment and communicates in a private language or at a preverbal level—requires a degree of patience and tolerance that is beyond the capacities or interests of most psychiatrists. Furthermore, it requires that the therapist not be one who insists on conducting all exchanges in an office at a set hour. These patients develop sudden accretions of anxiety that demand answering phones, providing extra appointments, visiting homes and hospitals at times to get over rough spots. With the borderline, ambulatory, or so-called pseudoneurotic individual, the initial relationship is less difficult to obtain, though it remains tenuous for a long time.

Today, the prescription of a phenothiazine must be recognized as a primary therapeutic move by the psychotherapist. Time has established that schizophrenics placed on such drugs function more effectively than others who are deprived. All should have such medication prescribed. Its administration allows reduction in affective arousal and its subjectively perceived intensity, its prescription establishes a bond between physician and patient, its ingestion demands responsible and regular observation.

An important aspect of the early stages of treatment of those schizophrenics who present a form of verbal contact that is incomprehensible to the physician is the necessity of working out the meaning of the patient's communications. In other words, a form of communication between the two must be established before treatment can proceed along more commonly understood lines.

Here one can discern a sharp diversion from the practices of analytically-oriented psychotherapy of the neuroses. The therapist does not attempt to have his schizophrenic patient associate, as if the patient were neurotic, to the verbalizations he is producing. Rather, he listens and tries to relate the verbalizations to the feeling tone of particular interpersonal events that are reported to have preceded the distorted communications or are observed to occur in close temporal relationship. Then, when particular communications are heard, the therapist may interpret the patient's feeling directly and make it possible for the patient to appreciate initially that he is understood and will not be hurt. Later the patient may be able to give up the symbolically distorted verbal communication for the more direct and customary modes of expression used by other people.

As an example, take a psychotherapeutic effort with a schizophrenic young woman who repeatedly ranted over Communism. She declared Communism was infiltrating the government, that our leaders were not cognizant of it and were paying insufficient attention to it. At the same time, she emphasized how early she herself recognized the Communistic threat, thereby intimating her superior powers of perception and interpretation. By careful observation of the sequence of events taking place in the therapeutic hours, it was noted that the outbreak of anti-Communistic ranting repeatedly occurred in relation to a series of associations in which she was reporting events in which she felt rejected, or when the psychiatrist's comments or activities suggested rejection. She was asked if she felt angry at such times and she admitted it. Subsequently, when the patient's vilification of Communism was observed, the therapist inquired what had taken place to arouse her ire. At such times she responded with a smile and immediately recounted some disturbing thought or event. It may be noticed that no effort was made to bring out an association to "Communism." It was assumed that her repetitive ranting in an angry way was related to some interpersonal action, either current or derived from the past, that aroused anger, and that the ranting provided a safe and symbolic display of the underlying emotions.

The same process has been evolved in resolving delusional thought in schizophrenic patients. Again, in contrast to the earlier psychotherapeutic efforts, the content of the delusion is ignored. Aside from the possible symbolic reference to interpersonal processes, the patient's remarks are listened to as a means of identifying their temporal relation to the train of interpersonal events taking place in the therapy, and their relation to similar disturbing experiences with others in the past. When it is clear from observation that the content is repetitively produced in connection with a particular interaction and its associated effect between the patient and others, an appropriate effort at clarification and interpretation is made.

Another clinical example may illustrate this point. In this instance, a brilliant schizophrenic young woman presented, as one of her original complaints, the somatic delusion that she had a body odor. No effort was made, nor any encouragement given, to have her attempt to associate to this symptom, to work out its origin, or to define its possible symbolic meaning. However, on the occasions when the patient reiterated this complaint, efforts were made, through questioning, to determine the actual circumstances in which she believed that she suffered a body odor. By "circumstances" was meant the time of the occurrence, the place, with whom she was associated and what the actions or words of other persons had been; and she was asked to describe these. It soon became clear that her somatic derogation occurred repetitively in situations in which she felt that someone toward whom she had some positive feelings made a move or gesture which she interpreted as rejection, and in which her loneliness was aroused. In examining each instance, it was evident that the patient responded in an oversensitive way and explained the behavior of others on their dislike of her "body odor." It became clear that the establishment of this thought was related to the passing of flatus in company—a forbidden and unmentionable act in her own family environment—which she had never consciously had the opportunity to discuss and learn about in the family circle. This delusion has its good point, "If I did not have body odor, they would like me."

At any rate, by defining the social setting of the expression of the delusion, it was possible to interpret on each recurrence the fact that the patient was speaking of another event in which she felt she was unwanted. The delusional expression disappeared, and she came to speak directly of her socially-aroused anxiety.

An important point in this therapeutic process is the continual alert appreciation by the psychiatrist of his own behavior in its totality and of its possible meanings to the patient. By necessity, the therapy is usually conducted with the schizophrenic patient facing the therapist. The patient has a continuing need to check his reaction through visualizing the gestures and moves of the therapist. The therapist must see himself as an active participant with his patient, and must be free to disclose his own feelings and the meanings of his actions in order to clarify the patient's frequent distortions of the situation.

Another departure from the customary analytic therapy of neuroses relates to the use of dream analysis. Most of those who attempt intensive treatment of the schizophrenic advise against the analysis of dreams. Work with dreams is considered unwise for several reasons. The most significant of these is that preoccupation with dream analysis perpetuates the patient's propensity for withdrawal into fantasy living. What such a patient needs, is to face continually the emotionally toned events of everyday living and to learn socially adaptive methods of accepting such events. Also, it is considered that the primitive impulses of such patients are evident enough in their overt pathology for dream analysis to provide little additional information. It is true that Lidz has recently suggested the usefulness of dream analysis in some schizophrenic patients in the later states of treatment. However, it would be unwise to disregard the long and hard-learned experience of many others, who have found that the use of dreams in treatment of the schizophrenic is more often harmful than helpful.

The psychotherapist must, in addition to his functioning as one who provides the source of a constant object relation from whom ego elaboration may proceed, must assist the patient in understanding the sources of his anxiety and in the reconstruction of his defenses. Such a psychotherapist has to be free to provide direct guidance and intervention in regard to aspects of social relations. He must assume, then, the responsibility for establishing the series of adjunctive aids that will lead the schizophrenic more certainly to perceive and accept his body as it is, to dare independent activities, to test trust, to support any initiative. He must assist actively any vocational or avocational interests without guilt, assist in developing more experience in complicated group social situations and in improving and encouraging efforts at self-expression. It is not surprising that Whitehorn and Betts have been able to associate social recovery of schizophrenic patients to the personal qualities of treating psychiatrists.[10] Such physicians have qualities of personal involvement . . . displayed in quiet competence, in periods of crises, attention to the relevant situational factors, willingness to personally intervene to assist the patients in accomplishment.

Much needed is a more thoroughgoing appreciation of the limitations of the psychotherapeutic process with the schizophrenic patient. Complete resolution of the schizophrenic process, fixed through ineradicable deprivations of early life, has not been obtained even by those with the greatest experience and patience. Fromm-Reichmann informed me that, aside from perhaps a single patient, she has not seen this aim attained.[4] Nevertheless, many enthusiastic psychiatrists press their patients beyond their capacity in order to reach the ideal. In certain instances incalculable harm is done by such therapists. There is a failure, often, to recognize that the goals stated by the patient are expressive of the wish-fulfilling aspirations of an ambivalently held parent. The talents of the patient are inadequate, the education toward the goal inappropriate or his motivation skewed by a thinly disguised hostile intent and lead to failure. Any failure ends with a further blow to self-esteem, usually coupled with regression and withdrawal.

Even more distressing is the meeting with schizophrenic patients who have been plunged into serious psychotic regressions when their therapists have severed the treatment bond in their own disillusionment. The willingness to recognize a continuing, supportive, though distant, therapeutic relationship without preconceived goals should be assumed initially in accepting responsibility for treatment of those with a schizophrenic illness. This step—which is realistic in the context of the experience of our profession at this time—provides in itself a significant forward move. By the continuing supportive role, it is the intent to signify only the willingness of the therapist to communicate with the patient periodically and when the patient indicates the need, after terminating the period of prolonged psychotherapeutic contact.

Let us now move to consider the evolution in therapy of the manic-depressive states. Here, too, we have evolved both a more sophisticated theory of the dynamics of their psychopathology as well as a major expansion in our ability to administer pharmacological agents useful in control of the differing affects and their related behaviors.

Psychodynamically, the cyclothyme is seen as one predisposed to profound affective disturbance through the actual or fantasied loss of a love object needed to maintain self-esteem. That object may be a significant person or a personal function or goal required symbolically to maintain the love and respect of the internally held significant human relationship. Predisposition, as a consequence of early deprivation in the parental transactions, though hypothesized, is far less supported by empiric data than for the schizophrenics. The manic depressive appears to have learned reasonably well in the family transactions ego attitudes of trust. His capacities for social conventions are well established, his desires for achievement and autonomy apparent, but are confounded by underlying sense of insecurity concealed by his ability to maintain a clinging dependency on others.

The loss brings about an infantile sense of hopelessness, with reduction of self-esteem and security, sadness compounded by varying degrees of anxiety, shame or guilt.

Such patients do not easily lend themselves, when retarded or hyperactive, to the rigid routine of the customary therapeutic process. The new efforts make it evident, however, that modified analytically-oriented psychotherapy is possible for some and seems beneficial.

The older failures raised a number of questions which have provided impetus for the new efforts. For instance, the clinical observation that certain patients treated by the classical technique became more depressed raised the necessities for understanding this fact psychodynamically and for modifying the technical approach to avoid such a complication. As mentioned, the depressive spell is precipitated by an actual or fantasied loss of a love object. The patient feels the loss as endangering his security. A depressive attack may sometimes recur on exposure to obscure symbolizations of such an event. As an example, the onset of a depressive period took place for one patient while she was doing some abstract painting related directly to cathedral windows, associated in her mind to a period of suffering during a trip abroad, made to abort the pain of a loss.

The initiation of psychotherapy, and for that matter, its continuing pursuit, is of an entirely different order with the cyclothymic than with the schizophrenic patient. While the transference relationship with the schizophrenic is one characterized by deep distrust and expectations of rejection, and is punctuated at times by explosions of hostility and accusations, the relationship with the depressed individual bears upon the therapist heavily because of the clinging dependency of the patient. The depressive patient demands that he be gratified. He attempts to extract or force the gratification from the therapist by his pleas for help, by exposure of his misery and by suggesting the therapist is responsible for leaving him in his unfortunate condition. He may offer promises or bribes as a means of attaining his dependency demands. Since these patients have learned well the ordinary techniques in social relations, their efforts are applied through means that are usually respected and are not easily put aside. Here, again, they differ from the schizophrenic, who is usually uneasy and inept in ordinary social relations.

Furthermore, the distortions of the therapist by the manic-depressive are in terms of a person open to the manipulations previously described or in terms of a moral authority, providing or denying approval, or in terms of a critical figure who fails to approve, but may indicate respect with acceptable behavior. This stereotyped distortion of the therapist, combined with the thought-retardation of the patient and the restrictive, repetitive associations, devoid for the most part of evidence of sensitivity for emotional interaction with others, requires of the therapist an inordinate degree of patience and little in the line of personal satisfaction.

Here again the therapeutic relationship is enhanced by the prescription of the appropriate drugs, whether it be a tricyclic compound for the depressive phase or a phenothiazine or lithium for the manic state. Such patients prefer to perceive their illnesses as constitutionally determined. Their shame is assuaged by the interpretation and the therapist may bring about both more secure contact with his patient and relief of the anxiety of responsibility by both stating the constitutional predispositions and prescribing medications—which supports the verbal opinion. Alleviation of affect, through the central effects of the drug, open communications with these patients.

Between the high personal standards that such patients usually have for themselves, and their feelings of impotence and incapacity, psychotherapeutic treatment may founder initially if the therapist urges productiveness. The patient's dilemma at this time appears to be of three sorts. He is unable to express the underlying sadness and rage that he feels, because of the guilt and shame which he attaches to the emotions of suffering. He expects that the expression of such feelings to the therapist will be met with lack of respect. Pressure by the therapist only arouses additional feelings of hatred and shame because of the patient's incapacity to meet the standards which he feels are expected by the therapist.

The program of therapeutic interviews on a four or five hour schedule a week is inadvisable. The demands of such a schedule provide an implicit insistence that the patient be productive, probably exaggerating his shame or guilt. The general consensus now is that depressed patients introduced to the psychotherapeutic process are better seen on one or two times a week. Furthermore, there should be no rigidity in requiring completion of the full therapeutic hour, if this seems undesirable. It may be mentioned that this variation of therapy protects the psychotherapist. The initial, if not the later, therapeutic sessions with depressed patients are incredibly trying to the therapist who must sit for long periods patiently doing little.

The writer has been personally impressed by the success of some psychiatric colleagues in the treatment of depressions. After some gross failures, applying the basic psychoanalytic technique in treatment of several patients with the manic-depressive syndrome, he found it useful to think of the differences between this technique and the techniques utilized by these colleagues. Without particular theoretical framework for treatment they utilized an approach which worked well in breaking through the depressive structure. Particularly conspicuous was the nature of the interpersonal contact with the patient, which was markedly at variance with the passive role of a psychoanalytic therapist. Two obvious features of this contact are worth comment. The first is the continual verbalized reassurance that the patient will recover. The second has to do with a certain directness and openness in dealing with the patient's problems. It would seem that these procedures fit into our present concepts of the needs of the depressive patient.

The patient is seeking another, or substitute, love object. The process of calm reassurance fits this need symbolically. The patient also has a need to escape from the feelings of guilt caused by his repressed rage in the depression. Consequently, in the early stages of therapy, whenever the patient has reported events which seemed to be conducive to the production of rage and anger within himself, but has left unsaid the emotional connotation of such events, the writer has personally adopted the practice of immediately verbalizing such feelings, and stating their relationship to other persons involved in the patient's situation. In this way the patient is relieved of the burden of stating his rage or anger and is not exposed to subsequent feelings of guilt for expressing these forbidden emotions. Yet he can identify the recognition of such feelings in another person whom he may respect, and, often, he accepts such remarks with a sly pleasure. With the use of this elastic, nondemanding, and at the same time active, interpretive approach, it has been possible to abort depressions in several patients; and also to supervise the treatment of young psychiatrists who have done the same thing, even for some patients who failed to respond to electric shock therapy.

Cohen and her collaborators[1] are also of the impression that the classical passive role of the psychotherapist is not conducive to success in treatment of the manic-depressive. They also warn against active rejection of the patient's demands as reinforcing his concept of himself as bad. Also, Jacobson[6] has pointed out that, in her experience, it is necessary for the therapist to show warm understanding, constant respect and an interest in the daily activities of such patients. She has advised that it is important to connect interpretations of the patient's transference fantasies with warnings of the future. The depressive patient's early good response is a spurious one; and, subsequent to it, the therapist may be confronted with the occurrence of a more severe depressive state or an elation. In the writer's experience, the therapist must be extremely alert to detect the recurrence of depressive aspects of symptomatology. Such a recurrence must be immediately related to its precipitating cause, either in current disturbances in the environment as an actual loss, or in fantasy of loss. Immediate interpretation has aborted the attack for several of the writer's patients on a number of occasions. Here again, it is necessary that the therapist be active in providing interpretation and taking full responsibility for doing so. Jacobson is also convinced that it is best initially to have the depressed patients focus on the experience of recent loss rather than on the earlier events in their lives which determined or reinforced their depressive symptomology.[6] With knowledge of the potential severity of the superego in these patients, it seems imperative that a cautious and slow psychotherapeutic introduction be used.

A consistently firm attitude is required to resist the inordinate demands of these patients. Experience seems consistent that, with relief of depression, they tend to wish to give up treatment. It is necessary to warn them of the dangers of too early detachment and that others have had recurrences or have been disturbed in other ways by premature withdrawal from treatment. Two patients followed by the writer over a five year period both had hypomanic attacks at points when they went on vacation (feeling well) or when they fantasied or imagined breaking off treatment with the physician. Both tended to deny the significance of their attachment to the physician and to derogate the value of therapy.

In the case of each of these patients, full commitment to treatment and willingness to work on the underlying interpersonal experiences conducive to the illness came about following the presentation of a dream. In each instance, the patient described bizarre dream objects to which he was unable to associate. When asked to draw the objects, one of the patients produced a simple breast-like structure, assumed to represent a mushroom, and the other drew a tractor wheel with a hub. The significance of these perceptions was immediately apparent to the patients, who had just been denying their dependent longings, with pseudo-independent acting out as escape from treatment.

In the treatment of patients with cyclothymic illnesses, the usefulness of dream productions and associations cannot be discounted. These cyclothymic individuals live a restricted life of fantasy. Through the association of dreams, it has proved possible to break through to deepseated associations which gave a clearer understanding of their basic longings and conflicts. It is worth remarking that this active use of dreams is in contrast with the avoidance of such material which has been noted in the psychotherapeutic treatment of the schizophrenic patient.

The effort to initiate psychotherapy for patients in hypomanic or manic states is even more complicated; but, with willingness to experiment, it has been successfully accomplished. Experience seems to show that with patients in these states—in which they identify with the covertly aggressive, sadistic and successful member of the family—the therapist must guard constantly against the provocation of rejecting a patient whose behavior seems designed for this purpose, as it is designed to embarrass the patient's significant object relations. In some instances, patients have become disturbed when therapeutic sessions were arranged daily, and, in others, the close contact with the physician has aggravated the hyperactivity, with relief occurring when the sessions were reduced. In most instances, direct firmness by the therapist has been salutary, particularly when dangerous acting out is occurring. Conversion of manic or hypomanic symptoms to the depressive is agreed to be desirable. It has sometimes been effected by the therapist simply indicating his doubts as to the soundness of the patient's presumption that he has reason to behave as if he were successful or in control of the situation.

An important source of conflict for the manic-depressive patient is that of strong hostility connected with envy which is repressed and avoided. In their series of patients, Cohen et al. found that the manic-depressive was often the best-endowed member of the family, and had been expected to provide the prestige for the group.[1] This position placed great responsibility on him, yet exposed him to the envy of his siblings, or even to envious competition with his parents. The future manic-depressive grew sensitive to envy and competition, and, to counteract them, unconsciously developed the pattern of derogating himself in order to conceal his full capacity. The writer's experience supports this opinion. The initial envious struggle appears to evolve in the Oedipal conflict.

The realistic aims of treatment of patients with the manic-depressive syndrome are to bring them to the point where they can consciously face periodic loneliness and separation without resort to submissive depression or revengeful overactivity. A real feat is the achieving of capacity to suffer a loss and be free of the pathological adaptation. Suggestive of such strength in the course of therapy might well be the patient's capacity to express his feelings of helplessness, sadness and rage directly and openly, and to expose his recognition of envy in himself and others. That these goals may be realized through a combination of modified psychoanalytic psychotherapy with appropriate prescription of drugs to modify extremes of affect is clear. My colleagues and I have maintained a number of patients in social homeostasis by such treatment. They never achieved through intermittent crises interventions provided during earlier phases of their illness.

In conclusion, you have been presented a point of view toward growth and development in psychotherapy. This point of view encourages and respects the continued need for technical experimentation and therapy revision. It emphasizes dynamic growth and sees stagnation in static reproduction. Perhaps the expressing of this point represents in itself the most important new look in psychotherapeutic evolution.

REFERENCES

1. Cohen, M. B., Baker, G., Cohen, R. A., Fromm-Reichmann, F., and Weigert, E.: An intensive study of twelve cases of manic-depressive psychosis. *Psychiatry* 17:103-137, 1954.

2. Frank, J. D.: *Persuasion and Healing*. New York, Schocken Books, 1961.

3. Freud, S.: Analysis terminable and interminable. *In* S. Freud (Strachey, J. Ed.): *Collected Papers*, Vol. 5. London, Hogarth Press, 1950, pp. 316-357.

4. Fromm-Reichmann, F.: Personal communication.

5. Hendrick, I.: Ego defense and the mechanism of oral ejection in schizophrenia; The psychoanalysis of a pre-psychotic case. *Int. J. Psychoanal.* 12:298-325, 1931.

6. Jacobson, E.: Transference problems in the psychoanalytic treatment of severely depressive patients. *J. Amer. Psychoanal. Ass.* 2:595-606, 1954.

7. Kiev, A.: *Magic, Faith and Healing*. New York, Free Press, 1964.

8. Kolb, L. C.: Psychotherapeutic evolution and its implications. *Psychiat. Quart.* 30:579-597, 1956.

9. Masserman, J. H.: Evolution vs. "revolution" in psychotherapy: A biodynamic integration. *Behav. Sci.* 2:89-100, 1957.

10. Whitehorn, J. C., and Betz, B. J.: Further studies on the doctor as a crucial variable in the outcome of treatment with schizophrenic patients. *Amer. J. Psychiat.* 117:215-223, 1960.

Acculturation, Language and the Secondary Process

HENRY W. BROSIN, M.D.

INTRODUCTION

I WELCOME THE OPPORTUNITY to discuss some topics I believe relevant to our work as practicing clinicians and/or behavioral scientists. There are no easy answers to most of the psychosocial problems which face us in our country, even when many of the economic questions recede into the background with current technological improvements in agriculture and engineering. We hope that, within a decade or two, we can provide at least adequate food, shelter and opportunities for more comfortable living for all of our disadvantaged citizens. However, it is a much more formidable task to educate a large majority of them to a level where they can compete with reasonable success for those values and symbols, including essential material goods, which give men both a sense of purpose and fulfillment in life.

With the growth of the "affluent society" and of organization man in our welfare state, it may be that property as such, or even children, will become less valuable as status symbols. Those who elect to compete in the hierarchy of power are becoming known as "meritocrats," and perhaps, as Peter F. Drucker says, this large and influential group of technical experts and professional managers will form a new voting bloc, and therefore a leadership rivaling labor, business and the farmer.[11] On the other hand, undoubtedly many other citizens not principally interested in the exercise of power, will choose other roads to fulfill their destiny, particularly as enforced leisure becomes the rule; and purpose in life and a sense of belonging to a community where one has identity, status, security, sympathy and love must also be available for those who do not live principally for the exercise of power. I am tempted to say that future administrators and managers must provide a meaningful community structure and activities for citizens who do not have them. I do not know if this is possible if the citizens concerned do not create their own community, as witness the sterile suburbs or artificial housing projects which seem to please very few after they are built. However, this seems to be a question which can be investigated in a

106

systematic manner and, therefore, of concern to behavioral scientists, including psychiatrists.

While some physicians remain dubious about the role of medical men in fields outside of medicine, as narrowly defined, in spite of the giant interlocking health programs with Federal and State agencies, industry and insurance companies, at the practical level, I believe most of us cannot avoid participation in socioeconomic and political activities, and many of us are being called on for leadership to provide the best possible care for our patients under existing conditions.

At the scholarly and investigative levels, physicians, particularly psychiatrists who have prepared themselves and earned the right to have considered opinions about large-scale social and psychological problems, have a responsibility to join the ranks of other behavioral scientists in trying to find new ways in which to help people live together in greater harmony. I would agree that uninformed psychiatrists have no special insights deserving of attention beyond that accorded other citizens.

We might take heart from the example furnished us by many leading physicists who, in their professional work are not concerned primarily with human relations, yet try to grapple with these problems. Niels Bohr, the father of the Copenhagen School and longtime dean of nuclear physics, did not need to explain or defend his essays on social and psychological problems, his principal interest during his last decade.[4,5] Similarly, Arthur Holly Compton,[8] Nobel Prize winner at Chicago who became Chancellor of Washington University in St. Louis, devoted himself to human studies, as did other notable thinkers, such as J. Robert Oppenheimer,[39] Eugene Wigner,[56] Isador I. Rabi and Victor Weisskopf, to name only a few of the more notable writers. Sir C. P. Snow wrote novels to illustrate psychodynamics which could not be written in essays, but are, in effect, case histories of moral and personal problems of scientists.

I believe it fair to say that the writings of my distinguished colleagues in this volume, Drs. Modlin, Braceland, Gerty, Farnsworth and Kolb, are highly concerned with values and their transmission.

DALLAS AND THE UNITED STATES IN 1917

It might be helpful to dramatize the differences between the decade during which Timberlawn Sanatarium was conceived and developed and our own decade by reminding ourselves of a few events of those horse-and-buggy days at the true beginning of the twentieth century (which really began with World War I) and contrasting them with the so-called "jet age." This will also help our imagination deal with the still dim and unpredictable prospects of the computer age now in the making.

I was led to this approach by a sentence furnished me by Dr. Talkington: that the original site chosen for the Timberlawn Sanatarium, "then known as the East Pike, was a half-day's buggy ride from downtown." I did not have the pleasure of knowing either Dr. James J. Terrell or Dr. Guy F. Witt, although I have heard many laudatory comments about them. I did know Dr. Thomas Cheavens during 1935-36 at the Colorado Psychopathic Hospital in Denver, where we spent many hours together one summer going over cases and theory. I want to pay tribute to him as one of the most remarkable men I have ever met because of his essential healthiness and solid good will. He had no hostility or ambivalence in his dealings with peers or patients. It was a pleasure just to be with him. I mourn his passing for several reasons, but one is relevant to this article, namely, we need to develop more men like him today in order to live better tomorrow.

While it is impossible to give more than a few of the stirring events, including World War I, and the new social and technological inventions of the decade surrounding 1917, I will mention some to illustrate the adaptations being made then. Of course, I should add that our writers in the early nineteenth century were also complaining of the increased tempo of daily living, alienation from the soil and basic values, so that we will need to specify our needs and goals to some extent to make them more meaningful. Dallas had grown from a population of 42,683 in 1900 to one of 158,976 by 1920.[50] There were 103 million people in the United States in 1900.[52] (There are almost twice as many now.[53] Dallas now has a population exceeding one million.) The transformations due to the motor car and good roads were just ahead. In 1915, Henry Ford had just started his uniform five dollars per day wage scale and the Adamson Act in 1916, establishing an eight hour day for railroads over the entire United States, had given organized labor its first major victory as a political force. Child labor laws slowly became more common and effective, and the vote for women was attained through the Nineteenth Amendment in 1920. The change of status of women in industry and business, of course, considerably altered family life and marital relations more than anything which has happened since. The new jazz music came into great prominence, and the new writing was now gaining public acclaim. It was indeed an axial time when new ways of doing things were becoming commonplace, and I need only mention the more general use of the telephone and the radio to come after 1922. Mass printing methods made cheap books and magazines much more available.

I should mention a number of legal innovations which are credited to Texas many years earlier because they are important social innovations unknown to most of us, although we live with them. "More important are the distinctive contributions of Texas to Western civilization: the union of the common and the civil law that produced the doctrines of community property and homestead exemption, the abolition of special pleading, and the blending of law and equity in a single court. These innovations, growing out of the Texas Revolution, have spread not only throughout the United States but to some extent throughout the English-speaking world."[50]

There is ample evidence that a relatively few highly placed citizens in Dallas are the major decision makers, and that they act in the best interests of the city, ". . . run it well, with self-effacement, not for private gain."[51] This raises the question of why men should act unselfishly and how this process can be initiated and nurtured. As you know, there are now calls made to the more prosperous members of cities to give a tenth of their time and energy to working on the race problem. Can our leaders arouse citizens, as we do in time of war, to give of themselves? Yet even in wartime, we find few men who say they are motivated by large abstractions. Most soldiers, particularly in battle areas, live for that small group of which they are members and which genuinely commands their deepest loyalties.

On the other hand, most of our social scientists support the ancient wisdom of the prophets and saints in emphasizing that for life to be meaningful it must have purpose, and that basically this purpose is the well-being of other people. The theme is familiar. How to implement it more effectively is our problem.

In this connection, questions are often raised whether man is infinitely adaptable to changing circumstances, and whether there are satisfactory answers given our present information. The point will be made in this paper that, while prediction is impossible and Utopias quite unlikely, given our present information as to the nature of man, nevertheless we need not admit total defeat even before we try as best we can to solve our problems. I cite the poet, T. S. Eliot, in his views on some aspects of the increasing complexity of life and art, in order to do justice to those who are burdened by modern tempo and organization: ". . . it may be maintained, the indefinite elaboration of scientific discovery and invention, and of political and social machinery, may reach a point at which there will be an irresistible revulsion of humanity and a readiness to accept the most primitive hardships rather than carry any longer the burden of modern civilization."[13] You will recall that Freud was also pessimistic on this score in one of his best essays, "Civilization and Its Discontents" (1930):

> The fateful question for the human species seems to me to be whether and to what extent their cultural development will succeed in mastering the disturbance of their communal life by the human instinct of aggression and self-destruction. It may be that in this respect precisely the present time deserves a special interest. Men have gained control over the forces of nature to such an extent that with their help they would have no difficulty in exterminating one another to the last

man. They know this, and hence comes a large part of their current unrest, their unhappiness and their mood of anxiety. And now it is to be expected that the other of the two "Heavenly Powers" (p. 133), eternal Eros, will make an effort to assert himself in the struggle with his equally immortal adversary. But who can forsee with what success and with what result?

I have taken time to review well-known material to emphasize the adaptations which all of us today have made and are now making in order to live in our increasingly complex world. Yet we have learned a few things since the first two decades of this century. Since those turbulent days, we have seen that monothematic social solutions such as "The War to End Wars" and "The War to Make the World Safe for Democracy" (1917-18), or "Votes for Women" (1920-28), or The Prohibition Experiment (1918-34), or child labor laws, or the eight hour day did not solve these problems, however valuable their intrinsic values may have been. I will name some of the more prominent current problems in order to establish the need for better basic information about how we can improve the current scene and teach our young to do more than merely survive at a subsistence level, economically or emotionally.

DALLAS AND THE UNITED STATES IN 1967

Most people think of nuclear warfare as our greatest threat, while others include conventional wars, both large and small, as highly destructive of our goals. Specialists in population and nutrition are certain that overpopulation is likely to cause the greatest damage to the United States and the world, and food experts are firmly predicting, on the basis of established data, that large famines are inevitable after 1976, and will reach enormous proportions after 1985.[25,40] Such events would affect the quality of life for all of us, and hence are conceivably also potential factors in determining the general and mental health of our citizens. With overpopulation come many associated difficulties, such as the pressures of overcrowding, excessive noise, pollution of air, soil and water, destruction of the natural resources, dislocation of people through various programs, and decline in quality of schools at all levels because excessive size often seems incompatible with excellence. Issues of birth control, including contraception, abortion and voluntary family planning; juvenile delinquency and crime, drug usage, racial rivalry and riots as a way of life; and scores of other manifestations of ignorance, injustice, poverty and prejudice will surely be emphasized and involve us all.

Both wars and increasing populations demand better global planning and more efficient centralized controls. I need not repeat the many warnings of our best writers on the evils of "Big Brother is watching you," as described by Aldous Huxley in *Brave New World*, George Orwell in *Nineteen Eighty-four*, B. F. Skinner in *Walden Two*, or Herbert Marcuse in *One-Dimensional Man*, among many others. The threats to personal liberty in these projections sometimes seem less hazardous than the decline of well-being, purpose in life and pleasure. The threat that a majority of us will be either unemployed in any meaningful sense or working in positions with relatively small responsibility and with increased alienation, anomie or spiritual malaise in the automated society, is held up as an even more destructive prospect by many social observers. Obviously, we are already experiencing these hardships with some serious misgivings and even pain, but as yet without total despair because we have developed numerous psychological defense mechanisms to shield us from daily information overload and a paralyzing guilt. Harvey Swados has recommended this "selective apathy" for problems about which the individual is impotent, but this does not, or should not, mean indifference at planning levels.[49] Most importantly, we have the hope, and confidence that with intelligence and massive effort we have the means and can acquire the abilities needed to surmount these difficulties, and many more which are to come. I would suggest, for example, that what Joshua Lederberg, the Nobel Prize-winning geneticist, calls "the ultimate scientific revolution: the precise control of human development," will be even more troublesome than most of our current problems.[30]

The evolutionary history of man suggests that ways will develop for him to survive even these onslaughts. Logically, we might be able to accelerate the processes whereby we can improve our condition, even though we are no longer naive about expecting to create a Utopia, because it is now more evident than ever that all systems are liable to error, and we are probably facing a long, long period of gradual amelioration of our worst faults.

THE HISTORY OF CIVILIZATION AS A GUIDE TO FUTURE DEVELOPMENT

Although prediction is impossible because of the numerous unstable variables, and the certainty of new and unpredictable technologic, biologic and psychologic inventions, I believe it worthwhile to study the history of civilization in order to gain as much useful information as possible to help us in our present crises. We can take some small comfort from the fact that civilized man, as we ordinarily understand the term, is a very recent newcomer on the evolutionary scene. While our physical apparatus has been developing over a period of one to two million years, our cultural history seems to be less than 50,000 years old at most, and even crude urbanization with agriculture and the use of domestic animals probably only 10,000 years old. Writing apparently came in about 5,000 years ago, but was developed only slowly over hundreds of years.[32,20,41] The Egyptians never developed a flexible fully phonetic alphabet, which was an invention of the Phoenicians around the tenth century B.C., and this discrepancy is only one of many which causes questions to be asked about the influence of the forms of language, and the way it is taught, because this may be a crucial factor in a developing civilization.

Since all of you are well acquainted with the evolutionary story of man's long journey from his animal beginnings, there is no need for me to even attempt a review. The recommendation that psychiatrists gain the time perspectives and historical insights furnished by archeology, prehistory and ancient history is an old one that was made by Freud (1926) and Adolf Meyer (1933).[17,35] Meyer said that psychiatry and neurology "should keep in advance of propaganda and not be the servant of it. . . . They deal . . . with functions laid down for an individual's entire life time. Its problems and solutions operate in terms of generations. . . . To integrate the thoughtfulness and the actual work on these extremes requires stability and a foresight of unusual scope. The progress of humanity depends on it."[35; p. 426] Meyer also stressed the interdisciplinary character of the study of man including paleontology, linguistics and semantics, and the evolution of language as bringing "us nearer to a history of psychology and of man-function than any other search."[35] These studies are essential for biologic understanding of integrated function in man, and also for the "control and use of his discriminating tool, with a better knowledge of both form and content of what may become available."[35] We have much greater need, but also much more usable data and methods for gaining useful information than when these words were written one generation ago.

While no one can expect psychiatrists to master the fields of archeology, linguistics, prehistory and cultural anthropology, it seems essential for them to have the minimal insights and perspectives needed to deal with the problems of acculturation of different races and classes both at home and abroad. Our educational systems, from the elementary schools through the professional schools, must redesign the curriculum so that it will deal with the study of man and his problems in a more realistic way, stressing biological, technological and socioeconomic factors so that all of our citizens may have a better understanding of how we are to combat ignorance, injustice, prejudice and poverty. To date, man's *adaptations* in biological evolution and his *adaptability* in social evolution have made him master of the earth. However, he carries within himself vestiges of both processes. Statesmen, humanists and scientists are increasingly aware of the dangers of man's uncontrolled or irrational impulses, and his meager knowledge of how to improve both the external and internal control systems. It is remarkable (in spite of many advances in social structure which should *not* be downgraded) that in many ways we have *not* solved the problems of intercity wars which occurred in early times in the Sumerian culture in Mesopotamia, or the Indus and the Greeks. The lack of balance between the forces of Dionysus and those of Apollo remains the central issue: man's conquest of himself.

I wish that time permitted me to review even briefly that "axial time" between 600-300 B.C. which is called the Golden Age of Greece, because here we can study those documents which show the tremendous growth in concepts and abstract thinking which characterize the best thinking in the Western World.[6,38,10,47,15] It is also a splendid introduction to the transition between thinking which is heavily weighted with primary process, and the partial ascendancy of secondary thinking, and could be used in this way in our curricula. This period and that described by Breasted as *The Dawn of Conscience* are the prototypes of what is needed in the coming centuries.[3] Less than five thousand years ago, men invented internal social controls, the steps for which can be read by any student. The coming of conscience as a social force must have been a tremendous event, even though it was and has been a less than perfect instrument. It would seem a less arduous task to perfect this device than our relatively crude ancestors faced in bringing it about in the first place. Perhaps our first lesson must be an understanding of how defective our personal standards and controls are. Emerson said it well: "We think our civilization near its meridian, but we are yet only at the cock-crowing and the morning star. In our barbarous society the influence of character is in its infancy" (Art of Politics).[3] I think Konrad Lorenz is credited with saying that we are the missing link between our primitive ancestors and Homo sapiens.

THE STUDY OF LANGUAGE

The origins and development of speech processes are very obscure due to the lack of physical residuals. Many inferences are possible from archeological evidence, and the many hypotheses include the importance of vocal signal systems to hunters, and to workers in clans and, of course, between the sexes.[22,23] The development of various dialects is an intricate subject which we can leave to the experts for the time being. There were few studies during the past five decades utilizing the evolutionary principle because it was considered speculative. This was doubly odd because the development of languages was probably the first solid chain of evidence that was available to biologists following the magnificent work of Sir William Jones (1746-94), English philologist and jurist; it made inevitable the study of the evolution of societies. Fortunately, the taboos introduced and maintained by the illustrious Franz Boas and his pupils, and also William James, seem to be lifting and younger men are again willing to deal with this difficult subject.[44] The lively debate on the differences between specific and general evolution and history is a welcome sign that cultural anthropology will help us better understand the transformations which are in the making as societies change from one form of operations to another.

The current ferment in the field of linguistics is so tempestuous that again I can only cite the experts and not attempt a summary.[1] For our purposes, some of these specialists are coming to grips with the problems of real men living in a real world, and have interesting observations and hypotheses about the adaptability of men in various cultures.

The newer studies for a neurophysiologic basis for language are also attempting to deal with the problems of memory and learning in man in an evolutionary manner relating brain to behavior in a fashion which is much more promising than older studies.[2,34,29] Lashley was most prominent in pointing out that not only is language one of the most important products of cerebral activity, however it may be related to the process of thinking, but that it also has organizational hierarchies which appeared to him as characteristic of almost all other cerebral activity. He was referring, of course, to the rational, conscious, secondary type of thinking. Lashley also pointed out that not only speech, but also all skilled acts involve serial ordering, including the temporal coordination of muscular contractions in reaching and grasping. He believed that analysis of the brain mechanism underlying ordered acts might ultimately lead to a solution of such complex problems as the physiology of logic.[29]

Newer studies utilizing elements from linguistics, mathematics, acoustics and electrical engineering to describe the communications process are also revealing. Linguistics is described by Martin Joos as being peculiar among mathematical systems, because physicists treat speech as telephony and describe it with continuous mathematics whereas linguists use a discontinuous or discrete system, such as a telegraphic structure. The larger units at the upper levels of communication deal with semantics; the smaller units at the lower levels deal with the phonetic quality where physicists work. Joos says that this is equivalent to defining a language as a symbolic system or a code.[26]

One interesting attempt to utilize a linguistic model of language to the psychoanalytic model of the ego is that of Miller, Galanter and Pribram.[37] They bring ideas from neurophysiology, communication and computer theory. Utilizing the concepts of Noam Chomsky, they attempt to estimate the size and complexity of what might be called the ego apparatus.[7] By analyzing grammar and syntax, they estimated how complex the planning device ego must be in order to generate grammatical sentences, and thus gain some lower limits for human planning equipment in general, nonverbal as well as verbal. Their analysis shows that earlier existing models for English grammar are not workable either for a child who must learn and use sentences, nor for an adult with a limited memory. These efforts are particularly meaningful because they present hypotheses which may be tested and thereby become useful to clinicians, educators or others who need such data in their daily work. They also stress the great value of studying grammatical systems as a method of investigating human planning. Grammar and human behavior are organized in hierarchical systems, and increased understanding of one helps understanding the other.

> The material is plentiful and relatively limited in type, it is easily described in writing, several alternative theories (that is, grammars) can be compared, reasonable intuitive agreement can be reached about acceptable and unacceptable sequences of responses, etc. With all these advantages, the scientific description of verbal behavior (by linguists, of course, not by psychologists) is far advanced over any other area of behavioral description and so provides a glimpse of what other behavioral theories may look like eventually.[37, p. 154]

Edward Sapir (1884-1939) probably deserves credit for a convincing demonstration that language as a total communication system is more than speech. In a series of brilliant essays relating language, culture and personality, Sapir influenced linguists and psychiatrists, through Harry Stack Sullivan, Margaret Mead and Clyde Kluckhohn, far beyond his professional circle.[44] In this brief survey, I can only recommend his essays to all psychiatrists who want to study the orderly relations between our communication systems, human behavior and social structure. The clinical demonstrations which I reviewed this morning are the best evidence that the intensive study of human signal systems will contribute to a better descriptive and dynamic understanding of human behavior.

THE SECONDARY PROCESS

The ascendancy of the secondary process first named and described by Freud (that is to say rational thinking as contrasted with wishful mythmaking) has been alluded to in relation to the development of conscience (5000 B.C.), and the development of abstract or conceptual thinking (5000 B.C.), and is familiar to all of us through Freud's writings on the ego and the id. Psychiatrists and psychoanalysts are confronted in their daily work with patients whose failures in living are attributed to the lack of internal control systems, rather than to some defect in the external controls. We have models for investigating these phenomena, and society expects us to help other behavioral scientists and educators to rear children more effectively to greater competence as cultivated human beings, and to help adults live together in harmony.

Of the many fascinating problems surrounding these questions, I will mention only two for your consideration. Benjamin Whorf (1897-1934) was a brilliant electrical engineer who became through his own efforts a gifted amateur linguist, and a pupil of Sapir following 1931 when Sapir went to Yale. In dramatic ways he revived the old problem of the extent and nature of the control of language systems over thought.[55] Ashley Montagu credits Giovanni Battista Vico (1668-1744) as the father of the new philosophy of language and mythology, i.e., symbol formation, as an early proponent of this thesis. Vico is more generally acknowledged as the father of modern history, cyclical theories of civilization and the forerunner of modern sociologic and anthropologic methods. This is not the place to debate the merits of the Whorfian hypothesis, which several eminent critics believe to be premature, poorly substantiated and misunderstood.[46,33,31,24,16] Apparently it is a subtle problem, with many facets deserving elucidation because of the implications for social control. For example, will more men practicing science, or trained to think and write scientifically, thereby become more "honest or honorable"? If we have more people with deep emotional ties to the motor car, airplane, learning machines and computers, will their attitudes on life become significantly altered, and, if so, in what directions? Aldous Huxley and George Orwell have taught us about "double-think" techniques, and "brain-washing" has been a common phenomenon in the past few decades, although these methods are crude compared to the controls with which the Whorf hypothesis is concerned. The Marshall McLuhan theme that "the medium is the message" comes to mind as another aspect. Philip Rieff, contrary to those men like Freud, Herbert Marcuse and Walter Kerr who see our civilization as threatened with increasing constraints, appears to believe that "the therapeutic attitude by many people will create a new morality in which the well-being of the individual and *not* the community will be the principal focus."[43] Obviously, much more than the forms of language and our total communications systems is involved, but psychiatrists are among the specialists who know much and could know much more about these trends, and can add to the sum total of knowledge needed to build a better world.

My second object in this section is to point out that, in spite of the tremendous insights written in many papers about the secondary process, in general psychiatrists and psychoanalysts have not developed linguistic theories of their own. Psychiatrists write many papers on speech, rituals, magic and art, but neglect some very interesting clinical leads. It is worthwhile to mention a book by a nonanalyst, Samuel Reiss, titled *Language and Philosophy* (1959). Reiss does not cite any of the Sapir-Bloomfield linguists, and does not apparently realize how close to Freud he is, in spite of three references to him.[42] In a notable review of this book, I. Peter Glauber, a New York psychoanalyst, makes the following comment:

> Why is it, language being the tool of the analyst—his daily bread, so to speak— that analysts have not moved beyond a mere few building blocks of their own toward a more substantial contribution to a psychoanalytic linguistics? We have quite a few germinal ideas which have not been sufficiently cultivated as, for example, some of Freud's concepts of regression in aphasia; the parallel of speech and ego development; Sperber's contributions on the relation of sexual events to the development of language; Kubie's body symbolization and the development of language; the contributions of Lewin and Bunker in relation to body-phallus and voice-phallus equations respectively; Fisher's work in relation to perception; the many contributions to the psychopathology of functional and organic disorders of speech. For those who think that these fallow areas need tilling, Reiss's study chould prove an inspiration.[49]

The immense amount of material in this area offered by Ernst Cassirer and his pupil, Susanne K. Langer, are further examples of possibilities. Cassirer gained worldwide fame for his studies on the correspondence between speech development and ego-formation without realizing apparently, until a year before his death, the similarity between his theses and those of Freud. Cassirer used psychiatric clinical material to good advantage from the clinic patients of Kurt Goldstein, many of whom were aphasic, with head injuries incurred in 1914-18.[46,28] He wrote at length about the origins of language, which were also the "dawn of a truly human mind."

There is one profoundly disturbing note in the dominant theme of the story of man's progress, slow but thrilling, to our present level of development, namely, that culture is a humanizing force, and that the cultivated *intellect* is indeed a guide to conduct. This faith has been taken for granted by most humanists and philosophers since early Greek times, until the wars and atrocities of the twentieth century called our attention to the fallacy of this position.[48] Many prophets are now aware that sheer intellect by itself may be trivial, as Bertrand Russell says, and may be of relatively little use in serious enterprises. The emotions and commitments in the hearts of men are paramount, even though we cannot live well without intelligent planning and direction of our affairs. Surely, psychiatrists have insights from their daily work with patients which can throw some light on how people are motivated and what value systems are most useful at this time.

WHAT CAN MEDICINE AND PSYCHIATRY OFFER TO EDUCATION?

Because I believe that education is the major medium for improving human relations at all levels, and our best hope for the near future—if we can avoid the major catastrophes of war and famine—I think it worthwhile to emphasize that psychiatry has something to offer the educational process. Dana Farnsworth has done an outstanding job in pointing out that we can teach the values of commitment, honesty and fidelity to the facts of how other people live and suffer; loyalty, tolerance and respect for all persons regardless of race, creed, color; perceptiveness for the needs and rights of others; sensitive awareness of one's own needs and wishes, including a knowledge of those qualities under one's control and those that are not; a proper humility and modesty with a proper balance between self-regard and a concern for the welfare of others; the ability to disagree with others without becoming angry, and without resort to force; the habit of inquiry and doubt; learning to live with ambiguity and uncertainty without passivity or paralysis.[14] Most psychiatrists would probably agree that the process of acquiring these qualities in the cultivation of an ego probably are a part of preventive psychiatry.

We have much to learn about the subtle dynamics of marriage and childrearing, let alone child development in a family setting, yet we also have much to teach from our clinical insights, and undoubtedly will do much better in the next few decades as our methods of investigation improve.

We have only begun to apply our insights to how people of all ages learn in various circumstances, and this field will become increasingly essential as we try to educate the underprivileged of all races in our own country. It is increasingly apparent that we are not well-equipped to educate the citizens of other lands, and, at this moment, many of our leading thinkers believe we are mistaken to try, except at the most basic technical levels of agriculture and industry. It may be useful to point out that many of our citizens, including our uncomfortable young, relatively small though their number may be, are essentially asking a single question: "Show us that it can be good to live in a democracy based on industry and technology and science. . . . If you only can show us that life can be good in the type of world you hold before us, it would give us great courage. Not only we but the entire world would follow you."[8] The usual replies are that many, if not most, Americans believe they already live rich lives, and are not overcome by feelings of lostness, alienation and tension; that working for their families, or for others whom they love gives purpose and meaning to their lives; and that there is always the hope for individual self-fulfillment according to the best of one's abilities. Of course, the latter is not available to all, but it is the American dream that young people cherish, and we can do our best to make it a reality for as many of our young as possible as soon as possible. To do so we must keep our own country intact and free from enemies until some method is found to stop wars between nations. This requires a strong defense. We also need a strong economy which will provide ample economic opportunity for all who can use it so that they can have jobs, housing, food beyond subsistence levels and, importantly, good health. We must do our share to provide health services on a broad base, taking care that the providing of health services does not impair medical research and teaching.

The problem of helping to define goals for the future is the most difficult of all, as it always has been in times of transition.[36,18,21,54] I have no ready answers, but will risk repeating what is well known to all of you, since it has come to us from the ancient wisdom; namely, that our ultimate goals will be defined by us as individuals, and that it is in our own hearts that we must decide what we want to be. This will not be easy, because most of us go along with the times, but we must endure the pain of complete honesty and candor in order to plan for ourselves, and for our children.

REFERENCES

1. *Biennial Review of Anthropology*, Vol. 1 (B. J. Siegel, Ed.). Stanford, Stanford University Press, 1959.

2. Brazier, M. A. B. (Ed.): *Conference on the Central Nervous System and Behavior; Transactions 1-3.* Madison, New Jersey, 1958-1960.

3. Breasted, J. H.: *The Dawn of Conscience.* New York, Scribners, 1933.

4. Bohr, N.: *Atomic Physics and Human Knowledge.* New York, Wiley, 1958.

5. Bohr, N.: *Essays 1958-1962: On Atomic Physics and Human Knowledge.* New York, Wiley, 1963.

6. Burn, A. R.: *The Lyric Age of Greece.* New York, St. Martins Press, 1960.

7. Chomsky, N.: *Syntactic Structures.* The Hague, Mouton, 1957.

8. Compton, A. H.: *Atomic Quest; a Personal Narrative.* New York, Oxford University Press, 1956, p. 335.

9. Dodds, E. R.: *The Greeks and the Irrational.* Boston, Beacon Press, 1957 (c 1951).

10. Dodds, E. R.: *Pagan and Christian in an Age of Anxiety; Some Aspects of Religious Experience from Marcus Aurelius to Constantine.* Cambridge, University Press, 1965.

11. Drucker, P.: American directions: A forecast. *Harper's Magazine,* 1966.

12. Ekstein, R.: Historical notes concerning psychoanalysis and early language development. *J. Amer. Psychoanal. Ass.* 13:707-731, 1965.

13. Eliot, T. S.: From Poe to Valery. *In: To Criticize the Critic.* New York, Farrar, Straus, 1965, p. 42.

14. Farnsworth, D.: *The Search for Identity* (The Edoardo Weiss Lecture, 1965). To be published by Forest Hospital, Des Plaines, Illinois.

15. Finley, J. H.: *Four Stages of Greek Thought* (The Harry Camp Lectures, 1965). Stanford, Stanford University Press, 1966.

16. Fishman, J. A.: A systematization of the Whorfian hypothesis. *Behav. Sci.* 5:323-339, 1960.

17. Freud, S.: *The Question of Lay Analysis* (1926). Standard Edition, Vol. 20. London, Hogarth Press, 1959, pp. 179-258.

18. Gabor, D.: *Inventing the Future.* New York, Knopf, 1964.

19. Glauber, I. P.: Book Review of "Language and Psychology," by Samuel Reiss (New York, Philosophical Library, 1959). *Psychoanal. Quart.* 28:548-553, 1959.

20. Grant, M.: *The Birth of Western Civilization: Greece and Rome.* London, Thames and Hudson, 1964.

21. Graubard, S. R.: University cities in the year 2000. *Daedalus* 96:817-822, Summer, 1967.

22. Hockett, C. F., and Ascher, R.: The human revolution. *Curr. Anthropol.* 5: 135-68, 1964.

23. Hockett, C. F.: The origins of speech. *Sci. Amer.* 203:88-96, 1960.

24. Hoijer, H. (Ed.): *Language in Culture; Conference on the Interrelations of Language and Other Aspects of Culture.* Chicago, University of Chicago Press, 1954.

25. Hornig, D. F. (Ed.-Ch.): *Effective Use of the Sea.* Report of the Panel on Oceanography of the President's Science Advisory Committee. Washington, D. C., The White House, June, 1966.

26. Joos, M.: Descriptions of language design. *J. Acoust. Soc. Amer.* 22:701-708, 1950.

27. Laffal, J.: Freud's theory of language. *Psychoanal. Quart.* 33: 157-175, 1964.

28. Langer, S. K.: *Philosophy in a New Key: A Study in the Symbolism of Reason, Rite, and Art.* Cambridge, Harvard University Press, 1942.

29. Lashley, K. S.: The Problem of Serial Order in Behavior. *In* Jeffress, L. A. (Ed.): *Cerebral Mechanisms in Behavior; The Hixon Symposium.* New York, Wiley, 1951, pp. 112-146.

30. Lederberg, J.: Some problems. *Sat. Rev. Literature* May 6, 1967.

31. Lee, D. D.: Linguistic reflection of Wintu thought. *Int. J. Amer. Linguistics* (Introduction), 10:181-187, 1944.

32. Life (Chicago): *The Epic of Man.* New York, Time Inc., 1961.

33. Longacre, R. E.: Reviews of "Language and Reality" by W. M. Urban and "Four Articles on Metalinguistics" by B. L. Whorf. *Language,* Vol. 32, 1956.

34. Magoun, H. W.: Evolutionary concepts of brain function following Darwin and Spencer. *In* Tax, S. (Ed.): *Evolution After Darwin,* Vol. 2. Chicago, University of Chicago Press, 1960, pp. 187-209.

35. Meyer, A.: British influences in psychiatry and mental hygiene (Fourteenth Maudsley Lecture). *J. Ment. Sci.* 79: 435-68, 1933. Also *in* Meyer, A: *Collected Papers of Adolf Meyer* (E. E. Winters, Ed.), Vol. 3. Baltimore, Johns Hopkins University Press, 1951, pp. 400-428.

36. Michael, D. N.: *The Next Generation; The Prospects Ahead for the Youth of Today and Tomorrow.* New York, Random House, c 1963, 1965.

37. Miller, G. A., Galanter, E., and Pribram, K. H.: *Plans and the Structure of Behavior.* New York, Holt, 1965, c 1960.

38. Onians, R. B.: *The Origins of European Thought About the Body, the Mind, the Soul, the World, Time, and Fate,* 2nd Ed. Cambridge, University Press, 1954.

39. Oppenheimer, J. R.: *Science and the Common Understanding.* New York, Simon and Schuster, 1954.

40. Paddock, W., and Paddock, P.: *Famine—1975! America's Decision: Who Will Survive?.* Boston, Little, Brown, 1967.

41. Piggott, S. (Ed.): *The Dawn of Civilization; The First World Survey of Human Cultures in Early Times.* London, Thames and Hudson, 1961.

42. Reiss, S.: *Language and Psychology.* New York, Philosophical Library, 1959.

43. Rieff, P.: *The Triumph of the Therapeutic; Uses of Faith After Freud.* New York, Harper and Row, 1966.

44. Sahlins, M. D., and Service, E. R. (Eds.): *Evolution and Culture.* Ann Arbor, University of Michigan Press, 1960.

45. Sapir, E.: *Selected Writings in Language, Culture, and Personality.* Berkeley, University of California Press, 1949.

46. Schilpp, P. A., (Ed.): *The Philosophy of Ernst Cassirer.* Evanston, Ill., Library of Living Philosophers, 1949.

47. Snell, B.: *The Discovery of the Mind: The Greek Origins of European Thought.* Cambridge, Harvard University Press, 1953.

48. Steiner, G.: *Language and Silence: Essays on Language, Literature, and the Inhuman.* New York, Atheneum, 1967.

49. Swados, H.: *New York Times.* August 31, 1967, p. 30.

50. Texas: *In: Encyclopaedia Britannica,* 1967 Edition, Vol. 21, pp. 891-901.

51. Thometz, C. E.: *The Decision-Makers: The Power Structure of Dallas.* Dallas, Southern Methodist University Press, 1963.

52. United States Bureau of the Census: *Historical Statistics of the United States, Colonial Times to 1957.* Washington, 1960.

53. United States Population: *In: World Almanac and Book of Facts.* New York, New York World-Telegram (etc.), 1967, p. 321.

54. Waelder, R.: *Progress and Revolution; A Study of the Issues of Our Age.* New York, International Universities Press, 1967.

55. Whorf, B. L.: *Language, Thought, and Reality: Selected Writings.* Cambridge, Technology Press of Massachusetts Institute of Technology, 1956.

56. Wigner, E. P.: *Symmetries and Reflections.* Bloomington, Ind., Indiana University Press, 1967. [Re: Biotonic Laws (Elsasser).]

The Value of Consultation

LAWRENCE C. KOLB, M.D.

THE PSYCHIATRIC LITERATURE pertaining to consultation has a soothing, warm and ego syntonic quality—for the psychiatrist. It is largely concerned with the almost total experiences of the psychiatrist serving as consultant to specialty groups other than his own. These reports are of value as much thought has been given to the nature of consultation, its definition and its conduct. Thus, there are excellent discussions of the relationship that exists between the consultant and the consultee, the reasons for and functions within the process of consultation.

In his emphasis upon the importance of crisis situations as they relate to personality disorganization, Caplan[1] has defined the kinds of consultant situations in which the modern psychiatrist often finds himself. He has addressed himself to this task with the conviction that the majority of the potential programs proposed by the Joint Commission on Mental Health and Illness will have to be performed by professional workers who have little specialized training in psychiatry, psychology or psychiatric social work—that is, family physicians, nurses, teachers, clergymen, probation officers, policemen, welfare workers, etc. He and others have suggested that a significant proportion of the time and energy of mental health specialists should be focused upon assisting through consultation the efforts (therapeutic and preventive) to enhance the capabilities of these professional groups in the care of those with mental and emotional disorders. To him, a psychiatric consultation may offer clarification of the issues, diagnosis, interpretation or advice as to treatment. It is not the consultant's function to act as therapist or supervisor. As a consultant, he may add to the knowledge of the consultee, clarify the understandings between consultee, client and others, and make it possible for the consultee to function more effectively in the future when confronted with similar situations. The consultant's principal functions, then, in relation to management of a particular case, is to clarify the goals of treatment, the techniques required to achieve these goals and the methods that may be utilized. He achieves his aims by gaining full knowledge of the treatment situation and recommends administrative manipulation and coordination of the actions and functions of the various persons significantly in relation to the patient.

To Caplan, a consultant may focus upon: (1) the consultee's problems in handling a specific patient or client, or (2) the consultee's administration problem in initiating and maintaining a program in which the immediate goal of the consultation is other than assistance in improvement of the care of a patient or client. Thus, some consultations are treatment centered; others are to provide assistance in administration. Some are concerned directly (or at least seem to be) with improving the care of the patient or the program; others are utilized to assist the consultee in his personal relations with the patient or the management of a program. This range of consultant practices today does not fall within the experience of every psychiatrist, nor is likely to do so in the immediate future.

While Caplan and others have devoted much of their energies to analyses of consultation with members of nonmedical disciplines, I suspect that, in volume, the greatest area for psychiatric consultancy is with our colleagues in medicine. I do not include here as consultation the direct referral of a patient for treatment by a psychiatrist.

Most of these efforts have been on the contribution of liaison services of general hospitals. This function, well established for at least three decades, provides not only a most valuable service to patients, but also assistance to our colleagues in the other medical specialties. Furthermore, patient reactions to such consultations are generally favorable.[3] Also, when well conducted, such consultations bring to general hospital medical and surgical services clinical instruction in psychiatry for beginning residents and attending staffs in other branches of the specialty. Recently, Lipowski[2] summarized admirably the published material on consultative psychiatry in relation to medicine.

Psychiatric consultation services in the general hospitals encompass a much wider span in actions subsumed than that under the frame of psychosomatic medicine. In the Columbia-Presbyterian Medical Center, we quickly relegated the term "psychosomatic" to a minor role when we discovered that the medical services staff often failed to request needed psychiatric consultations from the psychosomatic service and, also, that psychosomatic consultants sometimes refused to accept responsibility for consultation if the patient was suffering from a reaction which was considered other than fitting the concept of a psychosomatic medicine. Thus, our service for the general hospital now is simply designated as the Psychiatric Consultation Service. The psychosomatic designation failed as a communicative device to express the functions of a service of psychiatry to medical and surgical colleagues in a general hospital.

Lest we find our humility dissolving as we contemplate our services to others, let me quote some thought provoking remarks on this aspect of our consultation work. The sociologist Smith, in describing the psychiatrist as the magical man in the medical profession, declares this role is most apparent in his functions in the general hospital where he is "likely, as a widely ranging consultant to be an outsider on other physicians and surgeons services." Smith also warns that psychiatrists are accused of "Imperialistic intentions of making medicine its adjunct" and their missionary zeal to educate others provoke medical men to push them back. These comments perhaps represent reactions to poorly conducted medical consultation services or responses to the personalities of a few. Yet they deserve notice.

In light of the very extensive preoccupation within our specialty on consultative practice with other specialists, it is remarkable that there exists an almost total lack of comment upon consultation within and between members of the psychiatric-psychoanalytic group. Yet at no other time can I imagine has there been a greater need for just this kind of consultation. On what justification may such a remark be made? The justification is founded solely on reflections emanating from the emergence of many new methods of treatment in recent years and our own ability in terms of education and experience to recommend or offer these therapies. Different capacities exist in administration of the various modalities of therapy between individual psychiatrists and psychoanalysts and the different private and public hospitals and clinics. The indications and contradictions of the many new pharmaceuticals have added an additional problem in their many side effects and complications.

These changes have come about so rapidly that we have now several practicing generations of psychiatrists, each trained to perform the specific therapeutic tasks primarily used in his decade of active learning. And, among these groups, there is a widely recognized difference between those specializing in psychotherapeutics and in somatic treatments. Among those predominantly practicing psychotherapy are psychoanalysts, psychobiologists, group and family therapists and, more recently, behavior therapists. Then we have those skilled in administering electric and insulin shock or the full range of the pharmaceuticals. Some have entered subspecialties concerned with treating behavior problems of certain age ranges—child, adolescent or geriatric psychiatry. Very few, if any, are sufficiently widely trained and experienced to be thought of as outstanding generalists. It is this great variation in skill brought about by the tremendous changes in our therapeutic armamentarium and our own increasing subspecialization that demands more frequent consultations between ourselves. We should and must recognize the strength and limitations of our individual knowledge and skills.

Consultants are usually selected for their experience and known ability to provide a capable clinical judgement on the particular issue requiring solution. If the consultee perceives that his therapeutic regimen is under question by a colleague or relative, he will wisely select as a consultant some colleague acceptable to them both who is adjudged by the doubtful patient or his surrogate to have the adequate knowledge and prestige to provide a firm and fair judgement.

While these remarks may appear gratuitous, I can assure you from my own experience that the decision to request a consultation from a colleague, his selection, and the willingness to accept the role of consultee are far from easy for many within our specialty. In the last decade, my experience suggests that interspecialty consultations are brought about less often as the consequence of a well thought through professional decision by the treating psychiatrists and psychoanalysts than should be the case. Too often, the interspecialty consultation comes about through the intervention of another physician (usually a knowledgeable family internist), relatives or friends. The motivations in intervention are, of course, highly variable. But the fact that the intervention takes place in this way indicates that the treating psychiatrist or psychoanalyst has not fully or immediately perceived the transactional field of his patient and comprehended its homeostatic balances.

Let us, for the moment, look at some data collected from my office regarding consultation experience. It so happens that the office to which I am attached, as well as my own training over time in psychiatry, psychoanalysis and neurology, provides a substantial opportunity for a consultee to utilize me in a number of roles. During the last twelve years, of the approximately 500 consultations performed, 12 per cent were referred by psychiatrists or psychoanalysts to obtain an opinion as to the appropriate treatment or the conduct of an ongoing treatment. In 60 per cent of these instances, the psychiatrists requested the consultations. Eighteen per cent of the consultation requests were initiated by an interested family physician or internist and, in another 18 per cent, by a family member. There were personal referrals as well. Of the total of referrals for evaluation of psychiatric therapy, 30 per cent were concerned with the issue of continuing or terminating psychoanalytic or intensive dynamically oriented psychotherapy.

The vast majority (84 per cent) of patients referred for consultation were in office treatment. The remainder were in hospital treatment. As a result of the consultation, patients were recommended to continue in treatment with the consultee in one third of the cases. Patients recommended to be treated otherwise were assisted in transferring to another therapist or were brought to reenter treatment with another therapist in twelve instances out of fifty-four. Twice recommendations were made to transfer from office to hospital treatment, twice to transfer from one hospital to another where special treatment was available, once recommendation was made for the patient to be separated from relatives and, in seven instances, patients referred especially for consideration for treatment of a painful condition by the consultant were accepted by him.

Regarding the last course of action, consultation does not (as Caplan has indicated) necessarily preclude the acceptance of the patient for treatment by the consultant. In those instances where he has special knowledge, special experience or technical abilities, these are usually recognized by the consultee as the reason for the request for consultation. (In my case, the special experience which led to recommendation of transfers of patients to the consultant largely had to do with complicated instances of patients complaining of pain and/or complicated problems of self-induced illnesses due to masochistic orientation of psychosomatic complications relating to central nervous system disease.)

As to the consultation process itself, little needs to be added to the well-known formulas in those instances where the consultee directly decides and engages the consultant. Here the reason for the request is stated and, usually, the case record is made available and opportunity provided for the consultant to personally examine the patient. But the psychiatric consultant has a task in each instance which must not be overlooked: He must ascertain the potential hidden motivation which lead to the consultation request. Most frequently, this is due to arousal of some anxiety in the patient or the circle of persons involved in his treatment and management. The consulting psychiatrist must then ascertain the range of significant interpersonal relationships of the patient and the influence of the ongoing therapeutic process upon that circle of interrelated individuals. He will request and interview such persons other than the patient and consultee when it seems advisable. He may suggest that such a person be given his recommendations as well, either personally by him or in writing.

The essence of psychotherapeutic understanding today is the assessment of the sources of anxiety for the patient and for the significant interrelated individuals. This means that the perceptive therapist will identify all of the ongoing important interpersonal contacts and, from time to time, understand and assess the flux in those relationships as the patients personality is modified in the course of the psychotherapeutic experience. This is, from my experience as a consultant, the most overlooked aspect of the therapeutic process as it relates to the treatment of patients with chronic neurotic or psychotic conditions. The therapists have failed to assess the potential for disruption of the personality function of other individuals by change within the patient or to identify the significant and important bonds between patients and other persons.

It is from this source that the majority of the consultations are requested when they do not come directly from the engaged therapist. These requests either are made directly by the person or come from a medical relationship which exists in his family, and result from the insistence of certain psychiatrists and psychoanalysts that they must not contact other members of the family or the rational treatment will be prejudiced. The treating person, in these instances, has failed usually to evaluate the intensity of emotional bond between the patient and the significant relations. Nor has he felt the necessity to establish for the other member of that relationship some means of support to express his emotional disturbance caused by the shift in the emotional balance of this small social system. With our current awareness of the cataclysmic effects the other partner may suffer, I am inclined to believe it is our responsibility to assure health to the partner of a patient even though the bond between the two is considered pathologic. We know enough of such breakdowns that we can prevent them.

In my experience, the request for consultation by psychiatrists or psychoanalysts has usually come from the wiser and more experienced members of our profession. They have the awareness of the social spheres within which the patient moves, have often perceived the bogging down of therapy, have not been convinced that the therapeutic process must necessarily be interminable, have the great vision to understand that patients may perhaps achieve a greater degree of therapeutic success if transferred to another therapist. These are the attributes of the great practitioners of psychiatry. They are the same attributes that distinguish the outstanding practitioners of surgery. The latter knows when surgery is indicated as well as when not to operate. They appreciate that there are times when to retain patients as their own and other times when those patients must be transferred to a colleague.

The consultation process becomes then much more than the giving of advice to the consulting psychiatrist. It requires the determination of the many interrelations existing between the consulting patient and significant family member as well as the experiences of the patient in treatment in the past. The attitudes of the therapist toward the current treatment situation must be ascertained. The influences exerted by the attitudes and economic pressures of parental figures must be brought to light. And, certainly, one must assess the existing pathology and the change in behavior over time in relation to treatment, exigencies of the external situation, as well as the basic personality problem.

Most complex are those situations in which the relationship between the consultee and consultant comes about only after and as the result of intervention by someone other than the consultee. This situation is undoubtedly less fraught with difficulty for the consultant when the consultee contacts him after the intervening party has put his problem before another psychiatrist who then recommends he advise of his wish for consultation.

In those instances when an interested physician and family members or friend has come directly to the consultant for advice on some problem if patient behavior, it has seemed best to advise the requesting person to obtain consent for consultation from the treating psychiatrist or psychoanalyst. Unfortunately, in such situations the consultee has achieved his position unwillingly. Frequently, he has a feeling that he is about to lose a patient in whom he has invested much of himself, and, in such circumstances is sometimes unwilling to recognize the right of the external relation to question his therapeutic endeavor and feels resentment toward those he considers impairing his efforts. It has not been an infrequent experience to be told that it is impossible to provide a written summary. From such response, one can infer much regarding the operation of the consultee's office or the existing patient-physician relationship.

Whether a report is available or not, consultation is certainly best done only after face to face discussion with the consultee. There are some consultants, both psychiatric and psychoanalytic, who conducted their affairs without direct contact with either party. Where direct interview cannot be arranged or a record is unobtainable, telephone conversation is immensely valuable. The attitude of the consultee is frequently conveyed in their comments on the therapeutic contact. There is a potential for gaining some impression of the wish of the consultee to continue to devote himself actively to treatment in the future.

While much might be said of the need to refer for consultation patients who fail to progress well with the somatic therapies, it is my intention to discuss particularly that group of patients who have been in dynamically oriented psychotherapy.

Usually such patients are brought to consultation to ascertain whether the treatment is progressing satisfactorily or should be terminated or entrusted to another member of the specialty. There were sixteen instances of this kind. Three had been seen only for some twenty-five visits, another three for fifty visits, and ten had been in treatment from 100 to 700 hours. For the latter group of patients, the request for consultation came in every instance from the treating physician; all these were recognized medical psychoanalysts. On all occasions, the request for the consultation was made either by the internist who had been contacted by patient or family member. The family member usually declared that there had been no observable change in the patient's behavior. On other occasions, there was a desperate claim that the relationship with the individual undergoing treatment had been or was being seriously impaired. In a few instances, the statement was made that the treating person was not concerned with the physical health of the individual. In those instances where family members were carrying a portion or all of the financial responsibility for the treatment, there were questions as to whether this responsibility should be continued, withdrawn or restricted. Other questions put to the consultant pertained to the professional competence and the technical skill of the treating psychiatrist and the appropriateness of the treatment modality he had chosen for the particular patient. Complaining parents or marital partners spoke of the cold rejection of the therapists if they had been able to contact him. None reported advice from the therapist to visit another psychiatrist, discussions of the effects of treatment on family relations or useful sources for such material.

As previously mentioned, the vast majority of patients were advised to continue with the treating psychiatrist as a result of the consultation. For the most part, consultations seemed to come about due to emerging strains in the homeostatic relationship between patient and a concerned person. In some instances, the therapeutic process had led to a more direct expression of hostile aggressive or assertive behavior than in the past, thus upsetting a longstanding pattern of dominance-passivity between the patient and the complaining individual. In other instances, more prolonged therapy had brought about a social distancing of the patient from the concerned person as the patient commenced to perceive the pathology in the relationship and failed to respond to it masochistically as in the past. In still other instances, a son or daughter moved away from a dependent parent of the same or opposite sex to assume a more mature relationship with a peer, thereby threatening the clinging dependency of the parent.

In all those cases where recommendations were eventually made for the continuation of treatment as a means of further enhancing the maturation of the neurotic patient through the evolution of a mature independence, one wonders whether consultation would have been necessary if the treating psychoanalyst or psychiatrist had been kept abreast of the effect of the burgeoning knowledge on the family as a social unit, had been perceptive to the internal homeostasis of the family and been willing to depart from the rigid strictures of psychoanalytically-defined therapy to initiate or even clarify for the anxious relative the course of his continuing the treatment and his expectations.

The types of problems that upset a family in the course of intensive psychotherapy have been well-known for several decades. Probably no one has provided a clearer and better statement of them than Lawrence Kubie in his book *Practical and Theoretical Aspects of Psychoanalysis*. That changing behavior in one family member may lead to disruptive behavior in another family member is a well-known clinical observation. In instances where this occurred, the consultation served a triple purpose: (1) it protected the patient and allowed continuation of an ongoing and useful psychotherapeutic engagement; (2) it protected the therapist in his relationship with the patient; and (3) it provided needed support to the involved relative, who in some instances was referred for assistance.

Perhaps the most common reason for suggesting transfer of a patient to another therapist rested upon recognition that the patient and the therapist had been engaged over a long period of time in a motionless and difficult therapeutic relationship. Usually the therapist described his patient as an extraordinarily fragile person who was attending therapy as a means of assuring for himself a continuing but needed root for his dependency needs. Confrontation of the patient with this interpretation was considered too dangerous and the suggestion that he might make better progress with another person was avoided in the fear of harming the social functioning of the patient and precipitating regressive behavior. What often went unrecognized was the countertransference position of the therapist, which usually amounted to a hostile dependent relationship sometimes compounded with a secondary economic interest. The consultant frequently was able to determine the nature of the patient/therapist relationship through accounts of the patient's recollections of the therapist's comments to him when he had raised the question of termination.

Most complex and difficult were recommendations of a course of action that would allow loosening of an existing therapeutic bond without impairing ego functioning for those patients who had achieved some degree of social improvement in the course of their treatment. In those instances where the therapist harbored a hidden but negative counter transference toward the patient, there was seldom much difficulty. A suggestion from the consultant that another therapist could be found, was usually grasped eagerly. The problem, then, was to effect the detachment of the patient from the reluctant therapist. In some instances, the patients transferred their hope to the consultant. Here firmness was required on the part of both the consultant and the consultee with insistence that the patient attend the recommended new therapist. In other instances, transfers were effected but only with difficulty until the treating physician had worked through his own distorted dependent perception of the patient.

In rare instances, recommendations for transfer to other therapists were made early in the course of treatment. Such recommendations were made only when there was clearly an indication of patient exploitation. As an example, I may mention the young woman who was required to travel six hours each day for six days a week to see a psychiatrist in a distant town. Obviously, this arrangement pursued over a six week period of time completely disrupted the patient's potential for vocational activity and was seriously disturbing her relations with her fiance and family. Her father, a wealthy broker, requested advice from an internist who, in turn, advised the consultation. Her residence was in a large eastern city which boasts of probably the largest number of medical psychotherapists in the United States. The patient did well when transferred to a readily available and extraordinarily capable therapist living within a few moments of her own apartment.

Recommendations that the patient be transferred from one to another hospital usually occurred in the case of adolescents admitted to institutions without programs for this age group. Others seemed indicated for adult patients whose acting out propensities worsened in institutions which did not have the staffing capable of offering appropriate therapy. The right of the patient to consultation needs emphasis. Its denial is exemplified by the following recent experience. The patient, a manic-depressive woman, had been seen in psychotherapy five or six times a week for the past six years, interruptions taking place only when she became so overactive that she failed to appear for her appointment. The patient's brother, a physician, was aware of the claims of effectiveness of the phenothiazines and the lithium salts in the treatment of manic states. He suggested a trial on these drugs at onset of a hypomanic episode. The treating psychiatrist informed the patient that he could not agree to the treatment nor to a consultation, would charge the patient while she was away and, furthermore, when questioned by her family as to his knowledge of the literature on the use of these drugs, he commented that he had no motive to read even within the area of his own special interests. Undoubtedly, patients and families distort the comments of physicians, but it seems unlikely that this report represents a complete exaggeration of the transaction between the treating physician, his patient and the concerned husband. If the report approaches the truth, it represents in the patient's psychiatrist an attitude that does little credit to the specialty or the profession.

But of even greater importance is the denial of the patient's right to consider other forms of treatment more efficacious for her treatment. Certainly, each adult patient has that right. Those of us who are given the very great and demanding responsibility of treating many patients required to live within the limitations imposed by a protracted personality disorder, should periodically initiate review of that treatment through the process of competent consultation. In the case of psychoanalytic therapy, such consultations might well be arranged in every case after three years of treatment.

These experiences and reflections upon consultation within the specialty raise the questions as to whether we should paraphrase St. Luke's admonition to his colleagues, "Physicians, heal thyself," as "Psychiatrists, heal thyself" through consultation and postgraduate education.

REFERENCES

1. Caplan, G.: Types of mental health consultation. *Amer. J. Orthopsychiat.* 33:470-481, 1963.
2. Gross, M. L.: *The Doctors.* New York, Random House, 1966.
3. Kubie, L. S.: *Practical and Theoretical Aspects of Psychoanalysis.* New York, International Universities Press, 1950.
4. Lipowski, Z. J.: Review of consultation psychiatry and psychosomatic medicine. I. General principles. *Psychosom. Med.* 29:153-171, 1967.
5. Schwab, J. J., and Clemmons, R. S.: Psychiatric consultations. 14:504-508, 1966.
6. Smith, H. L.: Psychiatry in medicine. Intra or interprofessional relationships. *Am. J. Sociol.* 63:285-289, 1957.

Ethical Issues in Psychiatric Practice

DANA L. FARNSWORTH, M.D.

PSYCHIATRY probably is more exposed to public scrutiny than any of the other medical specialties. Its purposes and practices are often not well understood. No other medical specialty has so many actual and potential relations with disciplines outside the fields traditionally associated with the art and science of medicine. Since psychiatry is so often concerned with total effectiveness of individuals, with wholeness, or with improving the quality of interpersonal relations, its practitioners are particularly vulnerable to criticism regarding their life styles and professional practices—i.e., their functions as arbiters of behavior and taste necessitate their being exemplary in these areas or else being considered hypocritical.* Thus psychiatric ethics are a subject of intense interest and scrutiny.

The APA receives many requests for its code of ethics. There is none available. The code of ethics adopted by the AMA is the only one governing psychiatrists. Various attempts have been made by representatives of local and national groups to formulate a code specifically for psychiatrists, but no code which is generally acceptable has been devised even though numerous attempts have been made.

It is not the purpose of this paper to present rules or "answers," but rather to examine some of the issues inherent in the practice of psychiatry—particularly those which are controversial or which most consistently arouse discussion or criticism by laymen. The latter should be aware that his work with people who are emotionally disturbed increases the likelihood of the psychiatrist's being accused of reprehensible behavior. The gross forms of misconduct of which psychiatrists (and all other persons) may occasionally be guilty are hardly subject to dispute once the fact of their occurrence has been proved. I will attempt to discuss some of the issues concerning which there are no objective guidelines but only strong opinions pro and con.

PROFESSIONAL COURTESY

The custom of granting professional courtesy by physicians to other physicians and members of their families is as ancient as the Hippocratic

---

*In fact, psychiatrists are no more arbiters of taste and behavior than any other responsible citizens.

oath, and has been honored very widely for many centuries. The advent of prepayment plans and forms of treatment which require large expenditures of time has called the propriety of the custom into question. So far as I am aware, there is no consensus among physicians that the custom should be eliminated. Many persons do believe, however, that its application to specific circumstances should be modified.

When long-term care is needed, as in some orthopedic conditions, injuries such as severe burns which require months of care, or long-term psychotherapy, the physician furnishing the care may be subject to considerable financial deprivation. In many medical centers, certain physicians become known as the "doctors' doctor" and may find themselves embarrassed by insufficient income or by the necessity of submitting bills for services rendered.

With regard to the practice of psychiatry, retention of the code in its strict form may result in hardship rather than benefit to many physicians and their families. The latter may hesitate to request necessary treatment for fear of using up so much of a psychiatrist's time. A new psychiatrist may establish a practice in a small city in which there is no other psychiatrist and soon have so much of his time taken up by patients receiving professional courtesy that he cannot continue, thus depriving everyone in that community of his services. Or a psychiatrist may choose not to go to such a city, because he can predict that such a situation will arise.

In an effort to stimulate widespread discussion of possible modifications of the custom of professional courtesy, Dr. Hardin Branch wrote an editorial for the American Journal of Psychiatry in which he cited two pieces of evidence indicating that the principle of professional courtesy, as it stands, is detrimental to the physician-patient relationship: (1) 87 per cent of those physicians responding to the Judicial Council's survey owned some form of health insurance because "they felt better when carrying insurance," and (2) more than half of the internists, ophthalmologists, psychiatrists, allergists and pathologists admitted to some hesitancy in seeking professional care for themselves and their dependents. Dr. Branch's conclusion was that

> there is need to reformulate the concept of professional courtesy in spirit and in substance, with the overriding consideration in mind that its essential purpose must be to facilitate and enhance the best medical care that can be rendered one physician by another. The reformulation must be firmly based on the proposition that no physician shall make service to a colleague contingent on payment and that such service shall be provided in a spirit of pride and gratitude that one has been selected by a colleague to render it. Other things being equal, however, reimbursement for services rendered shall not be considered improper or unethical. The method of reimbursement, whether by gift, insurance payment

or direct payment, shall be frankly discussed between the physician and his physician-patient and agreed upon to the mutual satisfaction of both.[7]

A few weeks ago, the Judicial Council of the AMA issued a new statement which represents a more liberal interpretation of the custom of professional courtesy than has obtained in the past. Professional courtesy was defined as a model tradition rather than a rule of conduct to be enforced under threat of penalty. The propriety of accepting third-party payments was reaffirmed so long as neither physicians nor others make a financial gain from an illness. It is the responsibility of each physician, and a matter for his own conscience, to determine to whom and to what extent he will allow a discount from his usual and customary fees. A physician need not be embarrassed to accept a fee when he offers professional courtesy and the recipient insists on paying. Illnesses requiring frequent and significant portions of professional time and effort may be charged for "on an adjusted basis," which presumably means by mutual agreement. Finally, when financial hardship is present, professional courtesy should always be extended without qualification to physicians and those members of their immediate families who are dependent upon them.[8]

These changes are similar to the changes suggested by Dr. Branch, and permit flexibility of interpretation not hitherto possible.

CONFIDENTIALITY

Acts of violence, e.g., the multiple homicides that have occurred during the last few years, bring into the open the conflict between the offender's right of privacy and the public's "right to know." When the former has no history of psychiatric illness, the problem seldom attracts professional interest; difficulties and misunderstandings are more likely to occur when the alleged offender has a psychiatric record or if a psychiatric examination is made after the offense has been committed. The Committee on Ethics of the APA has recently prepared a statement concerning the release of material obtained in psychiatric interviews which will serve as a guideline for all psychiatrists, although it was prepared especially for the psychiatrist working for an institution. This statement has been approved by the Councils of the APA and the ACHA, the Council on Mental Health of the AMA, and has been declared as entirely in accord with the Code of Ethics of the AMA.[4]

The main provisions of this statement are as follows:

A psychiatrist should never reveal, except with proper authorization or, if necessary, under proper legal compulsion, for example, a court order, confidential information disclosed in the treatment process to him by a patient. Consultation with one's own legal counsel may be necessary.

With authorization of the patient, a psychiatrist may release confidential information, *but the psychiatrist should understand his duty to protect the welfare of the patient.* Such authorization should be in writing and specify to whom the information may be divulged.

Without the authorization of the patient, a psychiatrist should reveal information only in response to proper legal procedures as provided by statute in the jurisdiction in which he practices.

When a psychiatrist is served with a subpoena to deliver psychiatric records to an attorney, he should resist such order until he has consulted with his attorney with regard to protection of the rights of the patient. Moreover, he should notify the patient or the patient's legal representative of the subpoena. Psychiatric records should be released only when absolutely necessary under law.

When, in the opinion of the psychiatrist, it becomes necessary, in order to protect the welfare of the patient or the community, to reveal confidential information disclosed by the patient (for example, when he believes that the future behavior of the patient may constitute a risk of future injury to the patient or others), it is desirable, where possible, to obtain the authorization of the appropriate person, such as the next of kin, legal guardian, legal counsel, or by order of the court. In emergencies, it may be necessary, and is ethically correct, for the psychiatrist to take action without such authorization in order to protect the patient and others by preventing the patient from carrying out a criminal act. An example of such action is emergency detention of the patient in a hospital under proper statutory authorization such as an "emergency" or "temporary" certificate.

In cases of persons who have been under psychiatric treatment and who subsequently become involved in spectacular public crimes or whose condition may constitute a threat to the welfare of the community, the confidentiality of records (other than necessary for proper medical treatment) should still be maintained.

With respect to administrative procedures in settings other than courts of law (such as may arise in colleges or agencies established under law), the same legal and ethical principles of confidentiality and privilege rule, namely, the contents of psychiatric records should be divulged only when authorization of the patient or other proper legal authority to do so has been obtained.

After the death of a person who has been under psychiatric care, the pertinent principle of medical ethics cited above still applies. The confidentiality of the patient's communications should always be maintained except when the release of information is authorized by the proper person (that is, the next of kin, the executor, etc.) or under proper legal compulsion.

In colleges, in governmental agencies, and in the medical departments of industrial organizations, etc., psychiatric records should be kept separate from other medical records and should always be safeguarded. They should never be made available to nonmedical personnel, nor even to any other physician without the knowledge and consent of the psychiatrist who has examined or treated the patient, or without the consent of the Chief of the Psychiatric Service when this is appropriate.

It is to be emphasized that on occasions it may be in the vital interest of the patient that confidential medical information obtained by the psychiatrist in the physician-patient relationship be made available to the other physicians who may be called upon to treat the patient and, if necessary, recorded in the general medical record. Such a situation occurs when the psychiatrist is informed by the patient of his abuse of certain drugs; in such a case the physician (who is not a psychiatrist) in the college infirmary, or in a hospital, may later be called upon to treat the patient when he has subsequently been admitted in an emergency due to the toxic effects of drug abuse. Knowledge of the particular drug involved may be of the utmost importance in the immediate treatment of the patient.

If release of a psychiatric record is demanded by the administration, the college health director or other medical director should consult with the appropriate members of the administration, including legal counsel for the college or organization, regarding maintenance of the patient's legal rights. If ordered by legal counsel to release confidential records, such order should be obtained in writing.

It should not be forgotten that when records of a person who has died, or who has committed a sensational crime, are made public, the privacy of relatives or friends may be violated by such unwarranted breach of confidence.

As to the release of information obtained by a psychiatrist in a court-ordered examination after an offense has been committed, the proper course of action has not yet been clearly spelled out. In a recent celebrated case in which the findings were subsequently published in a national magazine, as well as in book form, the magazine publisher raised two questions: Is a psychiatrist justified in disclosing the details of confidential interviews with an accused murderer? Should details be published in a general magazine? The publishers answered both these questions in the affirmative when they printed the article. The psychiatrist, however, has a different frame of reference than does the journalist. In this instance, a signed release was obtained from the "patient."

But there are still a number of issues involved. Does the written permission really alter the ethical situation? Does the financial return to the writers influence the decision to publish the case history in a lay magazine rather than in a professional journal? Does such a precedent make future examinations of this kind more difficult to perform, especially when the "patient" does not know what subsequent requests may be made of him? Should the content of such examinations be released only by a court order? Is the release of such material in accord with the present medical code of ethics?

ABORTION

The new AMA policy on therapeutic abortion has many implications that are relevant to psychiatric practice. In essence, the new policy is a modification of the Model Penal Code of the American Law Institute and does not directly reflect reaction to policies established by state abortion laws. This policy has been developed with respect for both those physicians and their patients who are opposed to therapeutic abortions under any circumstance and those who hold liberal views. It does not assume as valid the position that all abortion laws should be repealed and that patients and physicians be free to use their own judgment in such matters.

In summary, the new policy permits therapeutic abortion only when there is documented evidence that (1) continuance of the pregnancy may threaten the health or life of the mother, (2) the infant may be born with incapacitating physical deformity or mental deficiency, (3) continued pregnancy resulting from statutory or forcible rape or incest may constitute threat to the mental or physical health of the mother. Two other physicians, in addition to the patient's personal physician, must examine the patient and record a concurring opinion, and the procedure must be performed in a hospital accredited by the Joint Commission on Accreditation of Hospitals.[1]

Several questions at once arise which concern psychiatrists' participation in such decisions. What constitutes a threat to mental health? Does a patient's insistence that she must have an abortion (with explicit or implied threat of self-harm) constitute such a threat? How will the socioeconomic status of patients affect these decisions? Does an unwanted pregnancy in a 40 year old widow or divorcee who is the sole support of several small children call for a different decision than it would for a woman with no dependents?

The foresight of the Colorado District Branch of the APA in developing a code for psychiatrists is commendable. Following passage of that state's relatively liberal law concerning abortion a committee was appointed to study its application. The impossibility of hard-and-fast rules was recognized, and emphasis was placed on making evaluations as individual as possible and avoiding generalizations about any particular diagnostic category. A warning to resist undue pressure from parents or other relatives was also included in the report.*

In brief, continual study and evaluation of how laws are being complied with (with provision being made for correction of abuses if and when they appear) is essential for psychiatry to maintain favorable public relations. The various District Branches have a clear and present duty in this matter as new laws concerning abortion are passed in their areas.

When simpler methods of abortion are devised, especially those not involving surgery, new ethical problems will arise which cannot now be clearly foreseen, and they must be dealt with in terms of circumstances then prevailing.

Collaboration with the Clergy

Much progress has been achieved in the last two decades in the development of close collaboration between psychiatrists and pastoral counselors. In many parts of the country, a clergyman is the only professional person available to whom an emotionally troubled person may go for help. Even in those instances in which the troubled person encounters difficulties with the law or accepted social custom, and has not sought help directly, the aid of a minister or priest is frequently sought by relatives, friends or court officials in resolving the dilemmas that have been created. There is now widespread (though by no means complete) agreement in religious circles that clergymen can serve their parishioners more effectively if they have had some training or experience under supervision in the handling of persons in emotional conflict.

I know of no fundamental reason why religion and psychiatry should be in conflict. Although the two disciplines have many goals in common, their areas of specific interest do not overlap. Erikson's description of the purposes of psychology (including psychiatry and psychoanalysis) as contrasted to those of religion is concise and poetic as well: "Psychology endeavors to establish what is demonstrably true in human behavior, including such behavior as expresses what to human beings seems true and feels true. . . . Religion, on the other hand, elaborates on what feels profoundly true even though it is not demonstrable: it translates into significant words, images, and codes the exceeding darkness which surrounds

*APA News, August 1967, p. 25.

man's existence, and the light which pervades it beyond all desert or comprehension."[6]

Issues of ethical import do arise from time to time because of profound misunderstandings between individuals. Many clergymen still believe that psychiatry is basically antireligious and that psychiatrists who respect or are sympathetic to religion are the exception and not the rule. When seeking a referral for emergency cases they may ask for a psychiatrist of the same faith as the troubled person. The argument that one should seek the services of the most competent psychiatrist available, regardless of his personal religious beliefs (or the lack of them), is not persuasive when the clergyman knows of derogatory statements about religion and members of the religious that have been made by psychiatrists.

Obviously the beliefs and convictions of psychiatrists concerning religion are their own, and are of no concern to others. But when disparaging statements about religion and religious people are made in the name of psychiatry (or under circumstances in which this appears to be the case), the bounds of propriety have been exceeded. The late Charles Curtis was indirectly referring to an essential quality of a mature physician (or other professional person) when he said, "There must be some talent which the expert in a special field lacks when he talks nonsense outside of it and which enables the man who is not a specialist, and knows he's not, to make sense about what he knows little about."[5]

PUBLIC STATEMENTS

When an individual psychiatrist advances a psychiatric interpretation of controversial events or behavior, his doing so often results in justified criticism of the entire profession. That the practice, even on an informal social level, has its disadvantages is illustrated by a comment by Jacques Barzun of Columbia University: "The number of snap judgments and flatulent pronouncements that I have heard at social gatherings from busy psychiatrists would fill several volumes of their own proceedings. They 'interpret' every remark, trait, and opinion; they characterize public and private character on the flimsiest basis. They take words for deeds. . . . The Hippocratic Oath ought to have an additional clause: 'And whenever I am tempted to show off, I will shut up.' "[3]

However, when crimes of violence or other dramatic and "newsworthy" events occur, psychiatrists are often pressed by reporters for "diagnoses" or explanations of motivation. A psychiatrist may be greatly tempted to comply, particularly if he thinks his comments will serve an "educative" purpose. But a premature or misguided response can do more harm than none at all. No rigid principles exist, but the following guidelines (which were published in the American Journal of Psychiatry) are relevant:

1. If in doubt, do not comment at all.

2. If you decide to comment, then do it thoughtfully. Tell the reporter that you will prepare a statement and call him back shortly. Restraint should be the guiding rule in all contacts with the press, radio or television. Understatement is usually more effective than excessive approval or denunciation.

3. In major cases of national interest, one may refer the inquiring person or agency to the American Psychiatric Association office in Washington.

4. When a call is referred from the APA to a psychiatrist, he is free to render whatever opinion he considers proper. It seems superfluous to add that even then, no "diagnosis" should be given unless an adequate examination has been made and proper written authorization has been granted by the patient, or, if he is incompetent, by his next of kin or legal representative. Also, no psychiatrist can speak for the profession as a whole. Official statements are made only by the Council or those officers of the Association empowered to do so. Among the more than 15,000 members, there is an infinite variety of opinions about any controversial issue.

5. Reporters may be referred to pertinent published articles or monographs that deal with the issue under discussion.[2]

REFERENCES

1. American Medical Association: Policy on therapeutic abortion. *J.A.M.A.* 201(7):544, August 1967.

2. (American Psychiatric Association) Farnsworth, D. L.: The psychiatrist as commentator on acts of violence. *Amer. J. Psychiat.* 123(8):1002, February 1967.

3. Barzun, J.: *God's Country and Mine.* Boston, Little Brown, 1954, pp. 267-268.

4. Committee on Ethics of the APA: Position statement on confidentiality and privilege with special reference to psychiatric patients. *Amer. J. Psychiat.* 124(7): 175-176, Jan. 1968.

5. Curtis, C. P.: *It's Your Law.* Cambridge, Harvard University Press, 1954, p. 38.

6. Erikson, E. H.: *Young Man Luther.* New York, W. W. Norton, 1958, pp. 21-22.

7. Branch, C. H. Hardin: Professional courtesy: Our problem. *Amer. J. Psychiat.* 123(8):1004, February 1967.

8. Judicial Council of the AMA: *Judicial Council Opinions and Reports.* AMA, 1967 Edition.

The Private Psychiatric Hospital
II. Present Day Leadership and
Service Potential

FRANCIS J. GERTY, M.D.

THE PRIVATE PSYCHIATRIC HOSPITAL, regardless of its ownership and management characteristics, exists essentially for the purpose of rendering treatment service to mentally ill patients. The worth of this service is what advertises it to the world. It should do its best to insure that the worth is there. If it does this successfully it provides an example of leadership and becomes also an instrument for providing leadership training.

It is well at this point to consider what elements go into providing quality hospital psychiatric services and how the factors that influence management to provide such service may operate for or against attaining the ends in view. A somewhat oversimplified listing of these elements and of the factors that influence them in operation of the private psychiatric hospital is offered here to furnish the basis for discussion of service quality and leadership potential.

These elements of principle and practice are about as follows:

1. Legally and medically the responsibility for direction of treatment of the individual patient is that of his attending psychiatrist.

2. Basic program of the hospital must provide additional support for his effort to carry this responsibility through the provision of personnel and facilities adequate for the purpose.

3. The administration of the hospital must have the design and operation characteristics that will effectually give this support continuously.

4. Therefore, the knowledge, objectives and attitudes of the persons in control positions are of extreme importance.

5. The psychiatric and other professional staff working toward the objective of good psychiatric treatment must have status in the hospital and influence upon administrative operations. It seems elemental that this staff should provide basic treatment program design and participate in the decisions on personnel and facilities to carry it through.

6. Since private psychiatric hospitals are not all the same in resources, ownership and management characteristics but are seeking comparable

142

results in offering quality service to patients, it becomes necessary to examine the differences in the principal categories of hospitals to determine how they may still provide the desired quality of service.

7. We discern at least three chief types of private psychiatric hospitals from the viewpoint of how the hospital organization is related to the care of the individual patient by the psychiatrist.

a) Psychiatric unit in the general hospital (not to be discussed in detail in this presentation).

b) Private psychiatric hospital with full-time staff or major part-time staff assuming all responsibility for treatment.

c) Private psychiatric hospital with visiting attending staff which assumes this responsibility plus some house staff members employed on full or part-time basis.

8. Considering private psychiatric hospitals from the viewpoint of charter of operation we find:

a) Nonprofit institutions.

b) Proprietary institutions.

9. The nonprofit foundation, as sometimes related to the hospital organization, is an adjunctive addition that will not be considered in this discussion but does merit study.

10. Programs of professional training approved by certifying agencies or boards are found in many psychiatric hospitals, but are considered here only incidentally as a good end to have in view after the basic ownership, management and treatment service relationships have been worked out in a satisfactory way. Their presence generally tends to give better promise of quality service.

The private hospital may be conducted as a proprietary one or on a nonprofit basis. Into which of these categories it fits does not of itself determine the quality of the service it can render. An ownership which takes pride in the excellence of its product and is intent upon keeping up that quality under the guidance of those professionally qualified to determine what constitutes quality may have a strong and direct influence in reaching the desired end. An ownership that resents such guidance or pays it lip service only while raising a host of specious objections for the purpose of maintaining a possessive control will never achieve quality service consistently in its hospital. There are many ways in which owners may throw their weight for or against the initiation and maintenance of quality psychiatric services. Whether they throw it for or against depends on how thoroughly they understand and how fully they accept the conditions that must apply continuously to provide the best possible standard of patient treatment in the hospital. That private ownership has been able to produce quality products in other fields is beyond question. When it does, the presumption is that it has followed the principles that experience indicates serve the purpose best in these fields. To provide quality psychiatric service also requires that the principles which govern the production of such service must be followed.

In a privately owned hospital the medical staff must be professionally well qualified, have status, and accept the responsibility for influencing the owners and administration to maintain the standards required to provide good treatment service. This applies in general to the medical director, his house staff assistants and the attending staff members. An item of great importance in securing this result would be the active support of a highly qualified board of trustees. Unfortunately, many hospitals that need this kind of support the most have great difficulty in getting and keeping it. Public spirited men and women, possessed of ability to render such service, dislike accepting it without sufficient assurance that the counsel they offer will be heeded. They must be more than figureheads or they will not continue to serve. Owners, finding board members more exacting than they had expected, may fail to use them or otherwise discourage them so that they will resign and be replaced by successors more amenable to owner influence. The general area of owner possessiveness resisting professional and policy-making specialists is one of the chief problems of the proprietary psychiatric hospital. Similar problems may arise in the nonprofit institution, but here the factor of possessiveness relates to something other than money investment: The avowedly dedicated man, too, may sometimes be inimical to good service operations.

The question may be raised as to how reasonable it is to expect that owners will accept such conditions as have been stated here. It is not an easy question to answer. Undoubtedly, the motivation which leads to ownership and the wisdom with which that motivation is coupled will have a good deal to do with what the answer ought to be. Unless there is enough wisdom to control it, the drive to possess may turn into a drive to sacrifice the basic objectives of service and gain power control or profit. This much is certain, if there is not understanding and acceptance of the conditions necessary for the provision of good psychiatric treatment service, consistently high quality service will not result. The hospital possessed by an owner so motivated may well survive, and even profit, because public need for psychiatric hospital service is great, but the survival will be at the level of minimum to mediocre standards of performance with regularly recurring anxiety about being approved at even this level when there is an impending inspection by a certifying agency.

It must be recognized that the members of the professional staff have a very real obligation to strive for excellence of service in the institution if they agree to accept appointment to it. This applies particularly to the attending staff, whose members treat patients in the hospital, and the medical director and his assistants, who are employed by it and who have day by day responsibility for the way the basic program operates. The duties which must be accepted to keep basic and specialized activities programs functioning well are numerous and time consuming and they do not become less so as the program improves. They are rewarding in their results not only in patient care but in the reputation which will come to the institution and its staff members. However, it is to be remembered that these possibilities of gaining credit for quality service must be dismissed if ownership and general management do not accept the conditions upon which quality professional service depend.

So far, only the conditions for the development of basic general program have been discussed and chiefly from the viewpoint of good in-patient care. Of course, the value of the hospital as a treatment facility can be remarkably increased by special additions to the in-patient service. Some of these additions have already come to be recognized as nearly essential in a psychiatric hospital of standing. High on the list is an out-patient service, particularly in visiting staff hospitals in urban areas. Community needs will almost require that some specialized service be supplied for adolescents and for children. Intensive care units, day and night service programs and family care programs are among the special programs most frequently mentioned nowadays. They will have the best chance of success if management has first effected organization of a good basic in-patient program with the necessary supporting personnel—psychiatrists, psychologists, occupational and recreational therapists, social service workers, etc. The in-patient operation must be both well designed and well controlled. If a hospital is to be worthy of bearing that designation a good in-patient service is the first consideration of all.

For promise of success in the proprietary hospital we must then expect

1. Ownership acceptance of professionally controlled standards of operation.

2. A board of directors and hospital executive committee of high caliber to set policy and authorize procedure in accordance with this principle.

3. A medical staff with leadership qualities that will have effective influence upon management to this same end.

4. A reasonable understanding of priority order in program development.

5. Realistic assessment of the financial feasibility of what is attempted.

Motivation in ownership has been mentioned. The owners of proprietary psychiatric hospitals may be of several backgrounds of experience. The profit motive may be the principal one and the owner may intend to be general manager as well as investor. Even so, the intention to render quality service may be an honest one. There can be considerable difficulty in getting an owner to understand fully the conditions which must apply in rendering quality service. It does involve relinquishing a great deal of management into the control of psychiatrically trained and other experienced professionals in the interest of treatment programs. The lay owner should fully realize and accept the implications of this. Proprietary institutions have been started not only by lay owners but by physicians specializing in psychiatry. Difficulties in the way of treatment program development may be fewer under a psychiatrist owner, but do exist. They are rooted in motivation, personality characteristics and administrative ability. The hospital may be in danger of becoming a one-man institution, though possibly a superior one. Inevitably, the day will come when the founder's vested interest will have to be transferred to a successor. The need for preparation for this event is obvious but doesn't always take place. Some excellent hospitals have come through this transition quite well, usually by converting to a nonprofit operation or to a partnership of owner professionals. Probably the best type ownership operation is one in which the owners are a group of psychiatrists who have common views of what constitutes good hospital psychiatry and who make provision for replacements in partnership to secure long-term continuity of this kind of service.

It can be granted that a proprietary hospital under the management of a single owner, whether layman or psychiatrist, if he is wise enough to learn what is required to sustain high standards of service, may attain these standards and flourish wonderfully. As has been stated, the day will come when this ownership and management must change. The history of private psychiatric hospitals is filled with examples of defunct institutions which were truly ascendant in their day. Many of them were often of the single or limited ownership type. Perhaps, even, the survival rate is greater with those institutions that have aimed at profit rather than high professional standing in their field. It is much more difficult to achieve excellence of service on a self-supporting basis than it is to survive with material profit while complying with the minimum acceptable standards set by inspecting agencies. We do not have statistics on this as yet. Governmental inspection agencies are increasing their requirements and, even more so, the nongovernmental agencies. These standards are set mostly by boards derived from hospital and medical associations. Insurance companies also insist upon value for benefits paid. It must be remembered that insurance companies are profit-making enterprises in the health field and proprietary hospitals could take lessons from them concerning the relation between maintaining standards of service and continuing in business profitably.

Keeping up the standards and continuing in business are the greatest tests that leadership must meet in the proprietary psychiatric hospital field. Since the service to be rendered is psychiatric, it should be expected that psychiatrists will be prepared to take a leadership position in this field. Otherwise they must be content to fit their contribution into a mechanism designed to serve a profit aim chiefly. We should not decry the fact that a profit aim must be included. Proprietary business must have more than a promise of profit to be continuously successful. We should decry diversion of most of the surplus of income over cost of operation into private pockets. There has to be guarantee of return of part of the profit, and a large part, to reinvestment in development of service. This is the matter on which success or failure of the institution and hence the success or failure of psychiatric leadership depends. That the progressive development of psychiatric service standards could take place without powerful influence from the profession of psychiatry would be a denial that a leadership role can be exercised by psychiatrists in determining the design and conditions of operation in their work in the proprietary hospital. If they hope to exercise such leadership, they must be prepared to do it. It will not be enough that they have a good background of professional preparation in their specialty, that they know how to treat the individual patient and what supporting hospital program activities should be provided. They must be prepared in the practical matter of holding their place in the hospital organization scheme. Only if they can do this will they be effective in securing the results for which they aim. To do so requires a knowledge of basic principles in administration and experience in solving the problems that continually arise in successfully carrying through programs that will provide excellence of service. Psychiatrists face a hard test if they work in the single or limited ownership type of institution. If they fail, they will become subservient cogs in the machinery, resentfully or resignedly grinding away at someone else's bidding. If they succeed, it will be greatly to the benefit of the institution they serve and to its patients.

There is not time to examine all of the types of proprietary hospital ownership which may be found and, therefore, the one which provides the simplest nucleus of organization has been chosen. This gives the clearest view of the inescapable problems encountered in attempting to ensure leadership toward continuously improving high goals of service with the focus directed upon basic ownership management relations.

There is a different and more complex pattern of ownership and management which seems to guarantee more certain progress toward the desired goals. This is the psychiatrist partnership owner type of proprietary hospital. We expect that the common professional background of the partners will obviate the need to educate the owners as to what is required for maintaining good psychiatric treatment standards in the hospital. The return of funds derived from profit to development should be less difficult to accomplish. Perhaps the greatest advantage possessed by this kind of ownership is the almost automatic operation of partner replacement with the passage of time to favor a vigorous and continuing growth. It makes less likely the occurrence of dissolution when key figures in ownership and management disappear from the scene. It is an important aspect of leadership that it be well aware of the need for replacement of key figures to provide continuity of excellent treatment service.

In this discussion it is taken for granted that internal matters of purely psychiatric design and operation should not be the principal objects of attention, but rather what environment may be provided for them in the proprietary psychiatric hospital so that they may best achieve their purposes. It is in its effect upon management that psychiatric leadership meets its greatest challenge in the hospital administrative field. The life or death of the proprietary psychiatric institution is determined by how this challenge is met.

The Psychiatrist at Sea:
An Illustrated Lecture on
Community Navigation

HERBERT C. MODLIN, M.D.

IN A CERTAIN CONGLOMERATION of humanity called Society, the geographic arrangement of the most populous region can be seen through the camera's eye as in Figure 1. Since I wish your attention focused chiefly on the cluster of offshore islands, only an area of the Mainland particularly relevant to my subject is represented. On the Mainland, a complex of imposing structures (referred to collectively as the Establishment) includes the numerous institutions of Government, Industry and the Military. The powerful Establishment, ruling through a system of benign oligarchy, has brought Society's general economy to fantastic levels of enterprise. Among the many beneficial and/or essential services available to the citizens of Society, I have chosen to discuss in detail these important few: Medicine, School, Church, Welfare and Penology.

The Medical People, living just adjacent to the Establishment, are exceedingly busy ministering to Society's needs. Of ancient lineage, theirs is a venerable tradition of magical prowess, rituals and secret passwords, and some tendency to aloofness from the Establishment. Indeed, through their administrative spokesman, known as the AMA, they occasionally quarrel with Government. Although their philosophy sometimes differs markedly from the Government's, they externally resemble the Establishment people, as exemplified by their magnificent buildings, the capital value of their investments in Industry, and their affluent way of life.

Church Island has been inhabited almost as long as the Mainland; its past fades into prehistory. Church Islanders and Medicine People have common ancestors; but the ancient tribe split into two factions and the schism exists yet. Church People are noted for their lofty moral preachments, worship of deities and concern with extramundane aspects of human welfare. Some of Church Islanders' forebears so militantly, so articulately held to exacting standards of conduct that a dissident ruling

Article reprinted by permission of The Menninger Clinic, Topeka, Kansas.

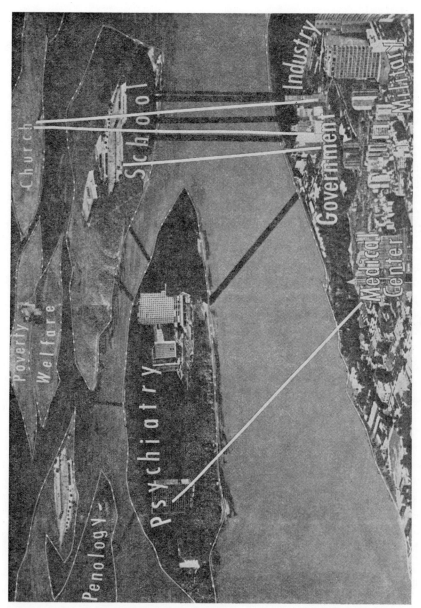

Fig. 1.

class expediently shipped them off to their own island. However, they are still highly esteemed; and to this day steady traffic flows between their island and the Mainland. But maintaining their insular separation from the bulk of population by a natural moat of surrounding seas appears a pacific arrangement, especially for Establishment people.

School Island is the most popular. Everyone in Society, with rare exceptions, spends some time there, particularly in his younger years. A flotilla of ferryboats operates each weekday. In recent decades, School has gained a considerable reputation as a youths' recreational resort; as a sitter-service facility to relieve overstressed parents; and (now being candidly recognized) as a mating playground. Starting at age five or six, children frequent the island in hordes; but, from early teens to early twenties, they tend to depart two-by-two, reminiscent of pairs debarking from Noah's Ark.

The atmosphere of Penology Island is gray, the living conditions constricted—a forbidding place where few go voluntarily. Those who must make the trip rarely benefit. Society, for the most part, is ignorant of and ignores Penology.

Farthest out is Poverty Island, another uninviting area. It has been explored and reports are that crops do poorly in the rocky terrain; that its natural resources are seemingly meager. Nearly all consumer goods are imported. Inhabitants observe odd local customs; and their argot is sufficiently unfamiliar, in contrast to the facile language of the Mainlanders, that intercommunication is difficult. It is a densely settled area and one of the best vantage points for studying a latter day phenomenon called Population Explosion.

The Mainland people express some sense of responsibility for the sad plight of Poverty although they do at times forget about it. You see, Mainland tries to be a happy place. Welfare Island has been set up as a distribution point and is a bustling port, indeed, these days. With its attained wealth, Society can afford generous impulses to honor some of its acknowledged obligations—an attitude particularly promoted by Government since new management took over a few years ago.

An additional tidbit of information culled from reports about this domain of Poverty: although the distance is the same and the obstacles one encounters en route similar, it seems much easier to get to Penology from Poverty than from the Mainland. The reader may consider this remark irrelevant; some of the Mainlanders think it irreverent.

Of the unparalleled social changes during the last twenty-five years, developments on the central island, Psychiatry, are not the *least* dramatic (Figure 2). The island's primeval forestlands have been partially cleared,

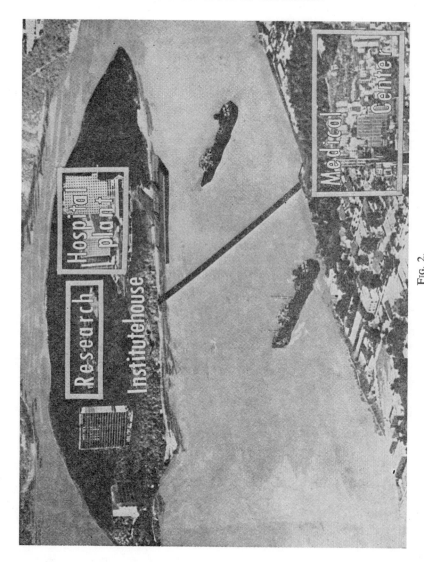

FIG. 2.

built up and occupied by a dedicated group of skilled artisans who emigrated from Medicine nearly a century ago and still loyally observe tribal customs of antiquity in common with the Medical People; but differences have evolved and strained relationships now and then erupt. Psychiatry's services are in such demand that traffic from the Mainland can no longer be managed adequately at the sluggish pace of ferryboats. A vehicular tunnel recently constructed to handle the crush is already in almost total capacity use.

On a central knoll of Psychiatry Island is Institute House, a manor of 19th Century architecture, erected when the island was a near wilderness. The original edifice is slightly dilapidated but structurally sound and some new wings have been added. Although certain critics think inhabitants of Institute House somewhat square, their work is respected and valued. They contribute to the economy of Psychiatry in a limited way through their fees for service to selected people from Society who need help, and some income derived from Psychiatry newcomers who pay for instruction in the mysteries of the Order. Many alumni leave the Institute to practice in various sectors of Society. The owners have been considering whether they might feasibly close the house and move to an office building in the island's City Center or even to the Center of Medicine on the Mainland. Meanwhile, the old manse is kept in a state of good repair befitting its distinguished historical influence. It is rumored that certain Institute members engage in a form of ancestor worship, but this has not been confirmed.

The largest building on Psychiatry (badly in need of modernization) is Hospital Plant. It employs many but needs more. Plans are underway to redistribute much of the Hospital's program to smaller branches in the vicinity of consumers—and to shut down part of the central plant.

As Figure 2 shows, much of the island has not been completely cleared or even explored. There is ample room for expansion. Most of the artisans have been so involved in providing goods and services that they have built up rather than out, seeming to prefer continuing their present lucrative and much appreciated practices rather than risking their time and energy on innovative ventures with unpredictable outcomes.

However, a small group called Researchers have been authorized to survey the frontier and seek to discover what creatures may be lurking in the deep forests, what latent resources may possibly be buried on the unknown side of the island. The intent and enthusiastic Researchers have been accepting subsidies from Government with which to purchase bulldozers, axes and divining rods. Many Psychiatry People are uneasy about this ingress of Government, but not sufficiently uneasy to devise alternate means for getting the admittedly important job done.

I must tell you that all on Psychiatry is not so well as it may seem. Dissatisfied with routine business operations, a restive coterie has voiced dissension. For several years, the malcontents have pored over maps, agitated for exploration of all areas of human habitation to search for whole new populations of potential consumers. They have published mountains of provocative material; have gained disciples rapidly; and their colleagues everywhere are discussing the pros and cons of this audacious movement. Government's vigorous backing and a crescendo of clamor for more services from the farthest reaches of Society are complicating factors. A phenomenal revelation: several members of the Institute elite have emerged from the manor to become leaders of the revolution!

Participants in the movement are not quite sure in what direction they wish to proceed or what vehicular means they will eventually choose for transportation. Illustrative of their quandry is the variety of names identifying the crusade: community psychiatry, social psychiatry, preventive psychiatry, public health psychiatry, comprehensive psychiatry. New as the endeavor is, splinter groups are already threatening to form.

Certain features are common to all variations on the new theme. One is a conviction that the good old days and the good old ways are not good enough when viewed in the perspective of a rapidly changing social order. Although we do admit that much is yet to be done on the island itself, including refinement of the helping procedures now in use; we recognize that we may be too uncritical of what we have been doing. In the rush to provide service, we take little time for painstaking evaluation of what our service accomplishes. While we have a pragmatic impression that most of our beneficiaries are satisfied (at least many of them refer their friends to us), we lack concrete evidence that our sizable outpouring of effort has effected much betterment in the community at large, since apparent and expressed need for service continues to exceed our upmost capacity through exertion of skilled manpower to meet it. The tunnel is clogged and a line of traffic, known as the Waiting List, is backed up well into the Mainland.

Much of a positive nature can be said about Society. It has achieved a high standard of living for a large proportion of its citizens, a high literacy rate, increasing numbers of college graduates, expensive and productive scientific laboratories, an exciting interplanetary space program, and a host of ingenious leisure time distractions. Coincidentally, it is squandering an enormous part of its gross national product and thousands of lives in a fruitless war on a faraway continent. Its statistics reveal shocking figures on homicide, suicide, highway carnage, venereal disease, alcoholism and drug abuse, divorce, juvenile crime, political scandals, racial uprisings, campus revolts, poverty areas and lengthy welfare rolls, and a numerically staggering incidence of prematurely disillusioned ("alienated") youth—these are among the less gratifying aspects of life in Society.

Depending on his bias and purpose, he who lives in Society might say "We never had it so good," or "We are sick, sick, sick." Obviously, both statements are valid within limits: social health and social illness coexist. Society is neither fish nor fowl—it is both; a hybrid monster of social evolution. Our historic past gives us few precedents for managing unique aspects of the present mass heresy toward the Faith of our Fathers and the traditions of our heritage.

Meanwhile, back at Psychiatry, our intrepid band of would-be explorers have a plan. They are going to sea. The progeny of generations of landlubbers, they intend to become nautically mobile; travel to all environs of Society, explore the needs for service, devise new methods of merchandising, and, above all, "Do something!"

No sooner is the plan announced than some of the newly initiated, action-oriented enthusiasts hoist sails. Many disastrously set out with inadequate equipment, obsolete maps and charts, and no training in seamanship. Some circle aimlessly in uncharted waters without making port, and some lose unseaworthy vessels in heavy seas, on submerged reefs. A few, having borrowed heavily from Government for the voyage, find themselves perforce working for their bureaucratic creditor in a job they had not anticipated and do not particularly like. Some resign from pioneering and return to the security of land, sadder but wiser for their brief adventures on the bounding main, taught by the failure of their impulsive excursions that they just happen to lack aptitude for a mariner's life. Back to tending their familiar gardens with zest and renewed vigor, they try not to mind echoes of "I told you so" from the island's more provincial stay-at-homes.

Despite setbacks, the Community Psychiatry group advances with purpose and optimism. Older experienced members lead this band of innovators in their serious and methodical creation of a worthy role. Utilizing the old ferry docks, they have set up training bases, have enlisted instructors and have devised a curriculum to teach boat building, command, navigation and cartography. A number of possible seagoing vessels and personnel are undergoing tests. Some small boats take a three-man crew patterned after the familiar three-man teams of artisans well known on the island for their diagnostic skills. A few large boats capable of huge payloads, now in the blueprint stage, will be manned by professionally qualified officers and a nonprofessional crew yet to be recruited.

The curriculum also includes all available information on the culture of populations to be visited and the characteristics of their major institutions. The basic needs of the prospective consumers are under scrutiny as well as new types of cargos and dockside loading and unloading methods. Special seminars, supplemented by field trips and tutorial instruction, present such topics as budget, logistics, grantsmanship, diplomacy, and the maintenance and operation of a steamship line.

Even such sober, organized efforts as these toward qualified maritime careers draw critical comments—"You are abandoning your prestigious professional role. You are, in effect, renouncing your citizenship."

Let us turn from the salt water analogy to less cumbersome, more straightforward language. The community mental health movement has been defined simply as "the delivery of adequate services to the consumer who requires mental health services." I decided to take this statement as the text for my sermon today, my exhortation to you, dear Brothers and Sisters, to turn from your past sinful ways, find the good life in community mental health, and give all praise to the Department of Health, Education and Welfare!

The statement stipulates "adequate services," a phrase which engenders an obsessional whirlpool in my mind. It suggests that services be delivered, but by whom? It implies consumers of the services: "those who require mental health services." I should like to discuss these three ideas in reverse order: the consumer, the deliveryman, and that intriguing phrase "adequate services."

1. Who is the consumer? Everyman? Many mental health professionals resist this uncircumscribed concept; but it must be considered. The community mental health movement constitutes only one aspect—in quantitative terms only a small aspect—of an extensive evolutionary change in American and possibly in world order. Notably, since the New Deal of F.D.R., we have developed and expanded socialistic concepts. Political scientists have recognized for years that ours is an era of creeping socialism. Certain obstacles and resistances emerging intraprofessionally in opposition to the widening sweep of the community mental health movement may actually be expressing a nonprofessional rejection of socialism.

It was indeed prophetic that our forefathers began the Preamble to the Constitution with "We, the people. . . ." At that time, the Federalists placed a restricted meaning in those words, a meaning consonant with representative rather than democratic goernment. That fateful idea is today being interpreted broadly by the Supreme Court, the President, and a compliant Congress to mean all the nation's people, regardless of race, creed, color or condition of pocketbook. As the struggle for a gaunt existence characterizes fewer lines in mid-century America, a second line of needs receives greater attention. Equal justice before the law shall be assured for all, including the poor; as shall be voting rights, education, individual enterprise and job opportunities. Current trends presage that the next "right" to be added to this list will be comprehensive medical service. If Franklin Roosevelt were President today, he might be championing a Fifth Freedom, freedom from illness.

Fifteen years ago, before the Joint Commission on Mental Health and Illness was conceived, an eminent medical sociologist, Leo Simmons, told a convention of the American Psychiatric Association that the natives were getting restless about morbidity and mortality. He observed an increasing discontent, particularly in the members of the lower socioeconomic classes, over the relative inaccessibility to them of widely publicized advances in medical knowledge and practice. Speaking for these medically underprivileged he said, "We mean to have it!" Twenty-five years before Simmons, Ortega y Gassett warned us of the inexorable *Revolt of the Masses* from political and cultural domination by a "superior minority." Hence, the consumer of mental health services may well be Everyman, and decisions more his than ours.

2. By whom shall services be conveyed to this composite consumer? Leo Srole, another medical sociologist, has characterized psychiatry as the public's court of last resort for many psychosocial problems. He suggests that when ordinary common sense measures fail to solve a social dilemma, increasing segments of the population turn to the mental health professionals, the experts in "uncommon sense." When the minister's counseling does not save the marriage; when the traffic court judges' fines and jail sentences do not deter homicidal speeders; when the school principal's persuasion and discipline do not stem students' incorrigible behavior; then psychiatrists may be asked to enter the arena. Should we respond readily? The pressure to do so is mounting.

At a recent meeting on Community Mental Health Administration, sponsored by the Council of State Governments and the National Institute of Mental Health, a legislator advised us how to "sell" politicians on providing mental health funds. Emphasizing that he was not interested in increased subsidization of traditional psychiatric clinics, he reminded us that the national divorce-marriage ratio is 250 to 1000; one divorce for each four weddings. In his state, the ratio is 336 to 1000, and in the county containing a metropolis, 552 to 1000. He declared, "If you can show us how to mitigate this social disaster or even just promise to work on it, you'll have no trouble in getting your mental health centers."

Challenges such as these, with dollar sign attached—are they subtle blackmail, an innocuous kind of bribery? Are we to become social scientists on the one hand, or assembly line marriage counselors on the other? Many of our colleagues are adamantly trying to hold the status quo, stay with the familiar in the face of multiple, diverse and novel demands on our time and talents.

How shall those of us, wishing to overcome our wariness of the "third revolution," proceed? Training and experience are advocated. At the Menninger Foundation we are retooling for a new training program in Community Psychiatry for third, fourth and fifth year residents, and have applied for an NIMH grant. The site visitor who came to check with us about our proposed program expressed surprise that we had not requested funds to extend our proposed training throughout *all* the years of psychiatric residency.

We consider it vital that the resident be trained first in dynamic psychology, hospital practice and intensive long-term psychotherapy to the point that he has a defined concept of the professional role of psychiatrist. We would recommend a similar order of preparation for members of other mental health disciplines. Once professional identity is familiar and secure, modifications and ramifications can be assayed with relative objectivity. Community mental health practice, which I view as a subspecialty, requires flexibility. Free translations of diagnostic and therapeutic functions from strict professional role definitions should at times be made. A well-integrated psychiatric team is able to perceive each patient or client as the team's responsibility, not just the psychiatrist's, and to assign necessary professional ministrations for the patient and relatives to whichever team members are most appropriately competent in the particular circumstances of a given case. This flexibility is best achieved through individual team members' yielding rather than arbitrarily maintaining their professional identities.

The value of experience in overcoming individual professional arguments against and resistances to practice in the community mental health movement has been well-documented. Regressive behavior characterizes some of the opposition: rationalizations, projections, denials, avoidances. I do not recommend plunging incautiously into this strange water; but, if we will but test it with one foot, we may find it not so chilling or deep or dangerous as we might surmise from the safety of the shore; and our initial "phobic" reluctance may be dispelled. The same swimming techniques which propel us easily across the heated pool may also keep us afloat and moving in the cold, shark-infested ocean.

3. Regarding my third point: what are the "adequate services" our conscientious but puzzled mental health personnel will deliver to a vaguely defined consumer? I have as yet in my own mind only a few convincing conclusions. The lightness with which this subject is touched in the literature suggests that my colleagues share my diffidence in tackling the uneasy and generally avoided question, "Isn't community psychiatry of necessity second-rate psychiatry?"

From one point of view, instant therapy for the masses seems called for. If, in responding, we spread ourselves tissue-paper thin, we may have to supplant the fifty-minute hour by the fifteen-minute exhortation; close the hospital ward, consign the patient back home to a neurotic spouse, and prescribe group therapy membership for him; view an exclusively private practitioner of psychiatry as socially obtuse, if not immoral. This Devils' Advocate position is not the only alternative; but outspoken defeatists and critics must be confronted. The phrase "adequate services" demands a value judgment and implies a standard measuring device, neither of which I can identify clearly at the moment. An obvious rejoinder to condemnations of "second-rate," that some help is better than none at all (first aid can stop the bleeding, splint the broken leg and counteract shock), will hardly reassure exponents of the pursuit of excellence. Perhaps it should not.

I hold that (1) a major research effort must be invested in our learning how therapeutic effectiveness is achieved and in discovering to what extent we do achieve it now, if we do at all, in our practice of both traditional and community psychiatry; (2) a glaring weakness of current therapeutic psychiatry is its neglect of adequate follow-up studies; (3) the best means to counteract the miasma of anxiety swirling above the vast swamp of community mental health matters is reality; solid firm reality, derived from objective scrutiny of ourselves, our practices, our patients' conditions and our cultural trends. Data from such scrutiny should give the lie to cynics who declare this swamp all bottomless quicksand; and should, as well, disconcert those who claim the swamp can expeditiously be drained sufficiently to support sound foundations for the next low-cost housing project.

Progress in the community mental health movement is handicapped by the overenthusiasm of much wishful thinking; by naive fascination with the new; and by an adolescent rejection of the old. We have been through these phases before—remember? In the beginning, two-thirds of schizophrenic patients were "cured" by insulin coma; sixty per cent of paranoid schizophrenics were improved by convulsive therapy; and similarly rosy results were initially attributed to psychoanalysis, lobotomy, tranquilizers, and a therapeutic milieu. Enthusiasm is not in itself bad: the new must be tested; be applied with mild indiscrimination; in a shakedown cruise be pushed to the limit that informs what it can and cannot accomplish, where its parts fit and where they rattle. *Furor therapeuticus* has value if perspective can be maintained and indulgence in chauvinistic adherence to an innovation can be resisted.

Undeniably, in existing community mental health programs, fog is prevalent. This is only one blurred spot, however, in the blanket of haze obscuring the visibility of reconnaissance into the tomorrow of societal change globally. Just where do we fit in? To us who will risk crossing over into the widening mental health frontier, it is becoming increasingly apparent that the established health-sickness frame of reference is no longer sufficiently comprehensive. There is a shift in emphasis—from treatment to rehabilitation; from symptomatology to social disability; from ego weakness to environmental stress.

My own search for clarification has led me to define community psychiatry practice on three levels:

1. *Psychiatric practice in the community.* In preparation for this modification of our traditional functions, basic instruction in general clinical skills is implicit. The existing public mental hospital, if a well-administered treatment institution, is a potentially valuable setting for demonstrating some fundamental principles of community psychiatry. The neophyte psychiatrist can learn to use this special community for the benefit of his patient; for example, he discovers how to (1) facilitate patient/psychiatric aide relationships, (2) utilize occupational therapy and industrial therapy assignments, (3) evaluate social work interventions with a distraught family, (4) clearly enunciate ward procedure which will be practicably understood by staff and patients alike.

Effective psychiatric practice in the community requires the adaptation of these clinical skills to community situations through the acquisition and promulgation of specific new attitudes and techniques; that is, basic psychiatric hospital and psychotherapeutic success are not enough for the effectual practice of clinical community psychiatry. Illustrative of this is experience gained from research at the Foundation which recently completed a four year study seeking to define and acquire the skills necessary for understanding and helping distressed low income families. Most of the personnel who participated in that research project are now staffing a demonstration and service unit within the Division of Community Psychiatry. This unit's purpose is furtherance and application of such knowledge and techniques as promise eventually to advance the effectiveness of professional help for malfunctioning families.

Among the intervention techniques our experience has proved valid, some are more in the nature of attitudes than specific actions. One attitude the project members found constructive evolved from their insistence on taking responsibility for a total family rather than for a single individual or for a limited family function (employment, welfare, health, education), which is *the* characteristic orientation of institutionalized agencies. Another attitudinal strength consists in a team's intentionally continuing, over a relatively long period, its helping relationship with a family burdened by various crises and chronic problems. Unlike many unifunctional agencies, we do not need to "close" a case once a single problem has been resolved. Teams express an essential professional attitude in being able to work intimately with a family and at the same time to avoid a position for or against either the family or any conflicting community agency.

The *ideal* aim of community support for faltering families is realized in helping the family grow, in stimulating the family's motivation to gain sharpened ingenuity in learning how to help itself. Through the promulgation and application of objective professional attitudes, this aim appears less "merely visionary" and becomes a more nearly attainable practical possibility.

The intervention techniques developed are several; a few will be described for illustrative purposes:

a. Functioning as clinical teams. A team of two professionals has charge of each client family: (1) to obtain two separate disciplines (e.g., psychiatry and social work); (2) to provide the mutual support needed by middle-class professionals entering an experience of "culture shock"; (3) to guard against a lone worker's dangerous personal overinvolvement in the multiple miseries encountered; (4) to provide a male-female factor which in certain situations might constructively serve as a surrogate parental model; (5) to facilitate communication with the clients. One common phenomenon of lower class culture is male-female role separateness. As an example, not infrequently men talk to men, women to women. After a team-family relationship has developed, the male professional may be talking to the male head of the family in the yard, while the female team member talks to the wife in the kitchen.

b. Visiting clients' territory. All clients are seen in their homes; none of the teams practice "office psychiatry." It appears necessary that the team make the overtures, see the clients in a setting most comfortable for them rather than for the team. Occasionally it is expedient to conduct an interview at the client's job, over a lunch counter, in a hospital, or in the team's car while transporting the client to his dentist or the court.

c. Defining the problem. By the second interview, the team usually has identified the presenting social complaint, as the family sees it, which allows entry of this team of strangers into the family environment and the family problems. The clients generally are action rather than verbal communicators; and the deep roots of many constructive relationships lie in early acts by the team to help with the leaking roof, the stalemated relationship between the family and a welfare worker, the family's confusion over the orders of the juvenile probation officer, or the procedure for getting the small child into Operation Headstart.

d. Hooking in. As just stated, many clients were in distress over their inability to find or negotiate with a community agency which might aid them. Often a team's interpretation of agency to client and client to client agency established a communication useful for initiating a helping process. Some clients are easily rebuffed and discouraged; some agencies are difficult to approach and penetrate. Frequently, misunderstanding and distortion occur on both sides which can be corrected by a knowledgeable intermediary. After the "hooking-in" process is accomplished, the team may be able to withdraw and turn to the next clients. In some cases, however the team must continue unobtrusive guidance of the family-agency interaction until optimal activation of the agencies' helping capacity appears assured or until the family learns how to get help on its own.

e. Holding interagency conferences. Individual agencies view conferences as expensive of staff time and rarely make communicative meetings a regular feature of their operations. Nevertheless, in many instances, teams have been successful in initiating conferences of representatives of the four, five or six agencies involved with a single family. Results may include (1) each conferee's increased awareness of the total family picture, and of where his agency may most contributively fit into the helping endeavor; (2) improved understanding of each agency's resources and limitations and problems; (3) a rearranged pattern of responsibilities and functions for helping the target family; (4) altered attitudes, diminished biases; (5) new ideas for intervention.

f. Supplementing the team's membership. In work with some families, the number on a team is temporarily increased by one or more special auxiliary personnel. A retired nursery teacher was introduced into one household where she demonstrated for the overburdened and ineffectual mother how one approaches small children. In another case, a skilled homemaker was enlisted to visit the client's home daily from four to six p.m. She showed the client how to (1) prepare well-balanced meals and (2) supervise and discipline her children when they descended upon her overwhelmingly after school. For still another family, high school students were engaged to tutor their junior high children in efficient study habits. These special "aides" do not replace the team but, rather, must receive regular supervision from the team for their maximal value to be realized.

2. *The Mental Health Consultant's Role.*

a. Many community organizations other than those staffed by mental health personnel, provide services for people suffering from psychological distress. Among these agencies are police departments, juvenile courts, welfare agencies, schools, health departments, adoption services, neighborhood houses and organized religion. It is widely agreed that psychiatric knowledge and techniques of intervention should be available as needed by workers in these agencies to the end that they may more ably conduct their stress-alleviating benefactions for clients. The mental health specialist's work in these agencies is usually termed "indirect" to indicate counseling with agency workers rather than directly with clients; he helps the "helpers."

b. The psychiatrist may indeed find himself "at sea" when he undertakes to adapt his clinical skills to a nonmedical agency serving nonpatients and operating within a non-health illness frame of reference. To function effectively, he must serve in "their" agency, learn their language, participate in their goal strivings and understand their problems. "Know thy agency" should be the consultant's First Commandment.

c. The Menninger Foundation's Department of Preventive Psychiatry specializes in the mental health consultant's role and renders this among other services through its various divisions and programs. Much department activity has developed in relation to major social institutions—law, religion, schools, industry and welfare—most of which touch significantly the lives of most people. The intent of these programs is prevention in a broad sense since all these institutions influence growth, development, adaptation and gratification in living. They may affect in varying degrees the psychological health and illness of large population segments.

3. *Administrator, Agency Consultant, Program Planner.* For careers exemplifying this highly specialized level of practice, postgraduate professional training and special aptitude and experience are needed. The number of practitioners is small, but the trend is toward increased interest on the part of psychiatrists and increased demand from the community. Psychiatrists are now functioning as directors of large, comprehensive mental health centers; as employees of and consultants to a variety of local, state and national bureaus and departments other than strictly medical; as consultants to urban renewal projects, Office of

Economic Opportunity projects and programs, broad rehabilitation efforts, etc.; as members of Human Rights Commissions, urban planning boards, housing administrations and public health research projects.

It is in this third level of community and/or social psychiatry that the medical role model receives its severest test, and "community navigation" is experienced by the clinician as fraught with reefs, cross-currents and gales. Here he must learn to deal with business leaders, fund raisers, legislators, accountants, politicians, bureaucrats, do-gooders and the raised eyebrows of his medical colleagues.

Basic psychiatric skills are essential ingredients for success in all these contributors to community action: psychiatric practitioners, mental health consultants, administrators and planners. There is persuasive logic in nominating mental health professionals for these responsibilities in that their standard technical proficiency provides them with sound approaches to fundamental psychological problems, whatever the setting. Some of the skills making them proficient pertain to the following:

1. *Interviewing technique.* Professional interviewing includes more than friendly conversation, information gathering, or even the establishment of rapport. It involves both diagnostic and therapeutic dimensions. Inexpert interviewing, particularly in the initial stages of an assistance relationship, can create serious obstacles to subsequent communication.

2. *Interpersonal process.* The well-trained professional has a sense of timing and process in interpersonal relationships: (1) an awareness that a relationship proceeds through sequential phases of development, (2) knowledge of how to guide that development, to shift adaptively as the quality of the relationship changes with changing circumstances over a span of time.

3. *Professional objectivity.* The professional comprehends the difference between empathy and sympathy; and his trained capacity to maintain relative uninvolvement of his own emotional vulnerabilities in the disabilities and misfortunes of clients is usually an asset. The professional helper's ultimate purpose is to lead and guide the client to a point of self-sufficiency that makes the helper no longer needed. Ideally then, the help given has an educational or maturational component and, at carefully determined times, the delaying or withholding of help is the most constructive move possible.

4. *Psychodynamics.* The trained professional, understanding the crucial influence of the irrational in human affairs, listens with "a third ear." He is aware of the importance of separating conscious from unconscious motivational processes; they must be handled differently. The basic prin-

ciples of human psychology apply to all interpersonal relationships; albeit many skeptics tend to deny the relevance of psychodynamics as behavioral determinants in people not labeled "patient." Whether the recipient of help be patient, client, offender, parishioner, job seeker, pupil or vagrant, he functions emotionally and mentally through common psychological coping mechanisms such as regression, resistance, avoidance, denial, projection, metaphor, substitution, displacement, transference, erotization and self-destructiveness.

5.*Growth and Development*. The discovery of handicaps or disability is only one of the problems approached by the mental health professional concerned with the several aspects of prevention, correction and adjustment. The helping task may consist in promoting growth in many clients of the lower socioeconomic income group rather than in trying to change an existing situation. Because of his theoretical and clinical knowledge concerning standard "normal" phases of growth and development in the human organism and the changing interaction of individuals and forces in their environment, he is competent to differentiate backward regression and arrested development. The professional, in contrast to the layman, should have a cultivated sense of the longitudinal life span and be alert to the possibilities for awakening and/or challenging latent growth potentials.

6. *Countertransference*. The mental health professional, through instruction and supervision, has acquired experience with countertransference phenomena, should know how to recognize them and how to get help, if needed, in using and controlling them. In short, he wears special eyeglasses for looking at both members in an interchange—the professional (himself), as well as the client. He has learned that the source of misunderstanding, misinterpretation and skewed communication may reside in either or both.

In the conflictual reality of our urbanized, bureaucratized and technologized social turmoil, the psychiatrist's role must be clarified. Adherence to the medical frame of reference, the doctor-patient relationship, the traditional diagnostic-therapeutic function, a splendid independence to select his patients—these may not henceforth be the psychiatric be-all and end-all. Psychiatry has been pushed toward and has, by its own option, moved toward a liaison position between medicine and society, a position analogous to that of a circus performer in the spotlight who rides around the ring standing astride two trotting horses. It is an uneasy position, especially if the horses are not pacing in unison.

The mental health professional, with his basic training suitably augmented, could become the "general practitioner" of applied psycho-social science. He appears the most available candidate at present—and if motivated to enlarge and remodel his traditional professional role flexibly to requisite training and experience—the one already best equipped to understand interacting, interlocking systems (intrapsychic, transactional, domestic, local, cultural). In addition, he is bred in a tradition of service and has a trained aptitude for intervention to produce change in the direction of successful social adaptation.

It has been said that the hallmark of maturity is the capacity to tolerate ambiguity and lack of closure. It has been said, also, that psychiatry in the broad sense is a young discipline. Undeniably, in community mental health programs, open-ended ambiguity is the current order of the day. It remains to be seen whether psychiatry, though young, is precocious, has attained sufficient maturity for the enormous task at hand. Perhaps in our rapidly changing professional scene the activation of a latent capacity in us to grow up in a hurry will be the most dramatic development!

Registrants

Adkins, Charles F., M.D., Beaumont, Texas
Adler, Justin H., M.D., Memphis, Tenn.
Altschuler, Milton, M.D., Houston, Texas
Alvarez, Luis A., M.D., Dallas, Texas
Anthony, Miss Louise, R.N., Portland, Conn.
Bailey, Walter H., M.D., St. Petersburg, Fla.
Bains, Louis W., M.D., Houston, Texas
Baker, David R., M.D., Dallas, Texas
Baker, Joseph J., M.D., Providence, R.I.
Bankhead, A. J., M.D., Tyler, Texas
Barbato, Lewis, M.D., Denver, Colo.
Barish, Julian I., M.D., New York, N.Y.
Bartemeier, Leo H., M.D., Baltimore, Md.
Bayles, Spencer, M.D., Houston, Texas
Beard, Bruce H., M.D., Oklahoma City, Okla.
Beavers, Robert, M.D., Dallas, Texas
Beck, Mortimer, M.D. (Capt. USAF MC), San Antonio, Texas
Bender, Nathan J., M.D., Shreveport, La.
Beyer, Alvin, Jr., M.D., Houston, Texas
Blair, James R., Jr., M.D., San Antonio, Texas
Blocker, W. Webster, Jr., M.D., Dallas, Texas
Bohannon, Richard F., M.D., Terrell, Texas
Braceland, Francis J., M.D., Hartford, Conn.
Brashear, Doyle S., M.D., Lufkin, Texas
Brener, Lazard S., M.D., Houston, Texas
Brien, Robert, M.D., Dallas, Texas
Brosin, Henry W., M.D., Pittsburgh, Pa.
Brown, Charles H., M.D., Wichita Falls, Texas
Brown, Hugh N., M.D., Terrell, Texas
Bruch, Hilde, M.D., Houston, Texas
Bullard, Dexter, M.D., Rockville, Md.
Bumpass, E. R., M.D., Dallas, Texas
Burns, G. Creswell, M.D., Compton, Calif.
Burris, B. Cullen, M.D., Chicago, Ill.
Butler, Charles F., M.D., Austin Texas
Cahill, Allen J., M.D., Dallas, Texas

Cantrell, William A., M.D., Houston, Texas
Carter, Dorothy, M.D., Dallas, Texas
Cassard, Lawrence J., M.D., Houston, Texas
Cato, Dorothy A., M.D., Houston, Texas
Charles, Henry L., M.D., Irving, Texas
Claman, Lawrence, M.D., Dallas, Texas
Clarke, Thomas P., M.D., Houston, Texas
Cochran, Winston, M.D., Beaumont, Texas
Coffey, Robert, M.D., Fort Worth, Texas
Cohen, Irvin M., M.D., Houston, Texas
Cohen, N., M.D., Hampton, Va.
Conners, Fritz, M.D., Dallas, Texas
Constantine, O. P., M.D., Waco, Texas
Cox, Virgil M., Jr., M.D., Fort Worth, Texas
Crank, H. Harlan, M.D., Houston, Texas
Crumley, Frank, M.D., Dallas, Texas
Daniel, Mrs. Diane, Dallas, Texas
Davis, Fred, M.D., Dallas, Texas
Davis, George W. Jr., M.D., Houston, Texas
Davis, Harry K., M.D., Galveston, Texas
Day, Kenneth, M.D., Galveston, Texas
DeBolt, Merlan, M.D., Dallas, Texas
DeFord, Horace A., M.D., Dallas, Texas
DeLoach, Asa W., M.D., Dallas, Texas
De Socarrez, M. L., M.D., Dallas, Texas
Dietz, Johanna, M.D., Dallas, Texas
Dimijian, Gregory G., M.D., Dallas, Texas
Dominquez, Florentino, M.D., Wichita Falls, Texas
Donahue, Hayden, M.D., Norman, Okla.
Donnelly, John, M.D., Hartford, Conn.
Dumonceaux, L. J., M.D., St. Louis, Mo.
Dyrud, Jarl E., M.D., Rockville, Md.
Easterling, W. S., M.D., Pineville, La.
Eckhardt, Richard E., M.D., San Antonio, Texas
Einspruch, Burton, M.D., Dallas, Texas
Ericson, Ruth Ann, M.D., Dallas, Texas
Erken, Ronald V., M.D., Wichita, Kans.
Eudaly, Harold B., M.D., Fort Worth, Texas
Ezell, Edgar, M.D., Fort Worth, Texas

167

Farnsworth, Dana L., M.D., Cambridge, Mass.

Fender, Tom H., M.D., Wichita, Kans.

Fisher, Albert L., M.D., LaCrosse, Wisc.

Ford, Hamilton, M.D., Galveston, Texas

Ford, Walter L., M.D., Waco, Texas

Frank, Thelma E., M.D., Corpus Christi, Texas

Frank, Thomas V., M.D., Waco, Texas

Frazier, Shervert, M.D., Houston, Texas

Freeman, Mrs. Betty, Cardiff, Calif.

Frenkel, Rhoda S., M.D., Dallas, Texas

Friedman, Carl, M.D., Waco, Texas

Fuller, David S., M.D., Dallas, Texas

Fullilove, Rowland E., M.D., Chapel Hill, N.C.

Gallacher, Paul, M.D., Shawnee, Okla.

Gerty, Francis, M.D., Forest Park, Ill.

Gilliland, R. M., M.D., Houston, Texas

Glen, Robert S., M.D., Dallas, Texas

Goodwin, Ben, M.D., Dallas, Texas

Green, Maurice S., M.D., Dallas, Texas

Green, Ralph S., M.D., Oak Park, Mich.

Grigson, James, M.D., Dallas, Texas

Hamilton, S. Sutton, M.D., San Antonio, Texas

Hansen, Douglas B., M.D., Houston, Texas

Hardy, Robert C., M.D., San Antonio, Texas

Hare, Henry P., Jr., M.D., San Antonio, Texas

Harrison, Robert H., M.D., Lewisville, Ark.

Haslund, Thomas M., M.D., Austin, Texas

Hauser, Abe, M.D., Houston, Texas

Hauser, Harris, M.D., Houston, Texas

Heatley, Maurice D., M.D., San Marcos, Texas

Herbert, Robert J., M.D., Dallas, Texas

Hibbs, Samuel, M.D., Tampa, Fla.

Hill, Al H., M.D., San Antonio, Texas

Hodge, Robert, M.D., Dallas, Texas

Hodges, Ralph, M.D., Dallas, Texas

Hoekstra, Clarence, M.D., Dallas, Texas

Holmgren, Robert B., M.D., Fort Worth, Texas

Horbaly, William V., M.D., Terrell, Texas

Huddleston, James E., Jr., M.D., Mesquite, Texas

Hughes, Ann, M.D., Dallas, Texas

Hughes, Delbert E., M.D., Dallas, Texas

Hughes, Waunell M., M.D., Dallas, Texas

Joliff, James, M.D., Waco, Texas

Jones, Granville, M.D., Summitt, N.J.

Joslin, Blocker H., M.D., Atlanta, Texas

Keller, Wayne F., M.D., Houston, Texas

Kennedy, Julien C., M.D., Marshall, Texas

Kimsey, Larry R., M.D., Grand Prairie, Texas

Kirby, Juanita, M.D., Dallas, Texas

Kleen, Juergen F., M.D., Dallas, Texas

Kolb, Lawrence C., M.D., New York, N.Y.

Kolb, W. Payton, M.D., Little Rock, Ark.

Kugler, Joseph S., M.D., Dallas, Texas

Kurth, C. J., M.D., Wichita, Kans.

Leaffer, Harry, M.D., Fort Worth, Texas

Leon, Robert L., M.D., San Antonio, Texas

Levin, Paul, M.D., Dallas, Texas

Lewis, Wade H., M.D., San Antonio, Texas

Linnstaedter, Celestine R., M.D., Houston, Texas

Littlejohn, Lake, M.D., Marshall, Texas

Long, Robert T., M.D., Dallas, Texas

Lorton, William L., M.D., Wauwatosa, Wisc.

Luton, Frank H., M.D., Nashville, Tenn.

McCauley, H. Leake, Jr., M.D., Fort Worth, Texas

McDaniel, Thomas W., Jr., M.D., Benton, Ark.

McQuire, H. Thomas, M.D., New Castle, Dela.

McNamara, Ray K., Ph.D., Dallas, Texas

McNeel, Tynus W., M.D., Tyler, Texas

Maldonado, Gilberto, M.D., Corpus Christi, Texas

Malone, James D., M.D., Fort Worth, Texas

Marshall, Mildred, M.D., Dallas, Texas

Martin, Jack, M.D., Dallas, Texas

Martin, Lawrence, M.D., Dallas, Texas

Mauk, Ferald D., M.D., Dallas, Texas

May, James S., M.D., Dallas, Texas

Meeks, John E., M.D., Dallas, Texas

Mendell, David, M.D., Houston, Texas

Menninger, Robert, M.D., Topeka, Kans.

Miller, William E., M.D., Dallas, Texas

Mitchell, Holland C., M.D., Waco, Texas

Mitchell, Mrs. Holland, Waco, Texas

Modlin, Herbert C., M.D., Topeka, Kans.

Moore, Kenneth G., M.D., Dallas, Texas
Moore, William Patrick, M.D., Houston, Texas
Moore, W. Taft, M.D., Dallas, Texas
Morrison, Bergen, M.D., Waco, Texas
Muirhead, Samuel J., M.D., Temple, Texas
Myers, Dan A., M.D., Dallas, Texas
Neiman, Richard N., M.D., Dallas, Texas
Nemir, S. S., Jr., M.D., Austin, Texas
Neumann, Charles P., M.D., New Canaan, Conn.
Nicolaou, George T., M.D., Dallas, Texas
Otto, John L., M.D., Galveston, Texas
Pack, John R., M.D., Fort Worth, Texas
Palasota, Pete, M.D., Abilene, Texas
Parker, Clarence R., M.D., Dallas, Texas
Pearson, D. B., M.D., Dallas, Texas
Peddicord, Orene, M.D., Dallas, Texas
Ponder, Jack E., M.D., Dallas, Texas
Phillips, Mrs. Austin, Dallas, Texas
Portman, Robert K., M.D., Dallas, Texas
Reifslager, Walter, M.D., Austin, Texas
Reitmann, John H., M.D., Dallas, Texas
Richmond, Julius B., M.D., Syracuse, N.Y.
Rigsby, Edith W., M.D., Shreveport, La.
Roberts, Gomer W., M.D., Irving, Texas
Roberts, Jean L., M.D., Irving, Texas
Rome, Howard, M.D., Rochester, Minn.
Rosenthal, Saul H., M.D., San Antonio, Texas
Rousch, Bernard, M.D., Hurst, Texas
Sable, Arthur D., M.D., Oak Park, Ill.
Scarborough, J. D., M.D., Waco, Texas
Schleuse, Louis W., M.D., Houston, Texas
Schuman, A. J., M.D., Dallas, Texas
Segal, Lester, M.D., Waco, Texas
Shadid, Ernest G., M.D., Norman, Okla.
Shelton, William P., M.D., Dallas, Texas
Shurley, Jay T., M.D., Oklahoma City, Okla.
Simmons, Belvin A., M.D., Dallas, Texas
Sims, H. M., M.D., Fort Smith, Ark.
Skinner, William M., M.D., Terrell, Texas
Slocum, Jonathan, M.D., Beacon, N.Y.

Smith, Charles L., M.D., Dallas, Texas
Smith, Charles M., M.D., Dallas, Texas
Smith, Claire, M.D., Dallas, Texas
Smith, Jackson, M.D., Hines, Ill.
Souda, Robert M., M.D., Dallas, Texas
Sparer, P. J., M.D., Memphis, Tenn.
Speakman, Walter F., M.D., Wichita Falls, Texas
Spier, Curtis J., M.D., Dallas, Texas
Stein, Paul G., M.D., Wauwatosa, Wisc.
Steindlu, Mr. E. M., Chicago, Ill.
Stevens, George M., M.D., Houston, Texas
Strickland, Sidney C., M.D., Pineville, La.
Stricklin, James L., M.S.S.W., Dallas, Texas
Stuart, H. James, M.D., Dallas, Texas
Stubblefield, Robert L., M.D., Dallas, Texas
Synor, Betty, Dallas, Texas
Talley, J. E., M.D., Terrell, Texas
Tejcek, Miss Elaine, Chicago, Ill.
Timken, Kenneth R., M.D., Dallas, Texas
Tripp, Larry E., M.D., Dallas, Texas
Vanderford, John, Dallas, Texas
Vogt, A. H., M.D., Houston, Texas
Waldron, Willard L, M.D., Jackson, Miss.
Walls, W. L., M.D., Pineville, La.
Watts, Maurice A., M.D., Lubbock, Texas
Webb, Robert W., M.D., Dallas, Texas
Weiner, Myron F., M.D., Dallas, Texas
Weisz, Stephen, M.D., Dallas, Texas
West, William W., Jr., M.D., Dallas, Texas
Wiesel, Carl, M.D., Lexington, Ky.
Weiss, Victor J., M.D., San Antonio, Texas
White, Paul, L., M.D., Austin, Texas
Whitley, Agnes, M.D., Dallas, Texas
Wiggins, Kenneth M., M.D., Richardson, Texas
Williamson, Edwin, M.D., Kalamazoo, Mich.
Willshear, C. C., M.D., Wichita, Kans.
Wolman, Walter, M.D., Chicago, Ill.
Woods, Ozro T., M.D., Dallas, Texas
Wright, Donovan G., M.D., Elmhurst, Ill.
Young, William O., M.D., Little Rock, Ark.

Timberlawn Psychiatric Center—The Medical Staff

Perry C. Talkington, M.D.
Charles L. Bloss, M.D.
Howard M. Burkett, M.D.
James K. Peden, M.D.
Jerry M. Lewis, M.D.
Ward G. Dixon, M.D.
Claude L. Jackson, M.D.
E. Clay Griffith, M.D.
Dode Mae Hanke, M.D.
Maurice S. Green, M.D.
Thomas H. Allison, M.D.
Stanley L. Seaton, M.D.
Doyle I. Carson, M.D.
Joseph W. King, M.D.
Keith H. Johansen, M.D.
Charles G. Markward, M.D.